100 BEST
Cannabis
Strains

100 BEST
Cannabis
Strains

A POCKET GUIDE
FOR MEDICINAL AND RECREATIONAL USE

Michael Blood, M.S.W.

Skyhorse Publishing

Skyhorse Publishing books may be purchased in bulk at special discounts for sales promotion, corporate gifts, fund-raising, or educational purposes. Special editions can also be created to specifications. For details, contact the Special Sales Department, Skyhorse Publishing, 307 West 36th Street, 11th Floor, New York, NY 10018 or info@skyhorsepublishing.com.

Skyhorse® and Skyhorse Publishing® are registered trademarks of Skyhorse Publishing, Inc.®, a Delaware corporation.

Visit our website at www.skyhorsepublishing.com.

10 9 8 7 6 5 4 3 2

Library of Congress Cataloging-in-Publication Data is available on file.

Cover design by 5mediadesign
Cover illustrations: iStockphoto

Print ISBN: 978-1-5107-5596-3
Ebook ISBN: 978-1-5107-5597-0

Printed in China

This book is dedicated to my wife,
Angel B. Hayes.
I am so very lucky to have her as my wife!

CONTENTS

KEY

SATIVA (s)
INDICA (i)
CROSS (Cr)
SATIVA DOMINANT (sd)
INDICA DOMINANT (id)

Introduction

With an ever-increasing number of states legalizing the use of cannabis (some requiring a doctor's prescription, others including for recreation), the buyer is faced with the question, "Which strain is going to give me the best results?"

This book is designed to answer that question and is in a format allowing the reader to carry it into a dispensary for a quick check of what can be expected with any given strain available therein. However, browsing through it, one is likely to find a good number of strains they want to experience over time and keep an eye out for.

While there are literally thousands of strains, there are the classics and there are the most recent and popular (both of which are likely to be available at any given dispensary).

This book will provide the reader with key information, such as:

- Sativa/Indica ratio (Sativa increases mental focus and even energizes, producing a "high" while indica strains sedate, relax the body, and impart a feeling of being "stoned." Hybrids attempt to provide the best of both.)
- THC levels: How strong is it?
- CBD levels: A key factor in many of the medicinal benefits
- Possible side effects: From Euphoria to Dry Mouth to Anxiety, and the percentage of people who experience them
- Medicinal benefits and the percentage of effectiveness in each category
- Taste and smell

- Growing information, such as flowering time, yield, and special needs

This and much more—for each strain.

Here is how to interpret listing for uses for medicinal and recreational, as well as any potential side effects:

- (ExH) 100% of users experience this effect to a very significant degree
- (VH) 80 to 90% of users experience this very strong effect
- (MH or HM) 70% of users experience this significant effect
- (M) 40 to 60% of users experience this very noticeable effect
- (LM or ML) 30% of users experience this usually mild effect
- (VL) 5 to 20% of users experience this mild effect
- (ExL) < 5% of users experience this usually very mild effect

Note that some effects may be listed without percentages. This is because that information was not available, it was was worthwhile to include those terms for potential users.

100 BEST
Cannabis
Strains

100 Best Cannabis Strains

Notes

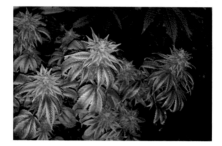

Strain: Acapulco Gold

Dominance: 100% sativa (Landrace, Mexico)
Parent Plants: Landrace
Grower: Wherever you can find it, but some "crosses" are out there (*not* Ac. Gd.)
Awards: *High Times* Cannabis Cup winner (sativa, 2010)
THC: 20–22%
CBD: Not reported
Flowering: 11 weeks
Yield: Medium
Potential Positive Effects: Euphoria (H), Pleasant (H), Relaxation (H)
Potential Negative Effects: Paranoia (VL)
Reported Treatment Uses: Alzheimer's (H), Pain (H), Spasms (H)
Description: One of the most popular strains of all time.
Growing Hints: Typical of sativas, the plant is a tall, robust grower.
Additional Notes: Beware some selling a cross they call by same name—make sure to get Landrace!

100 Best Cannabis Strains

Notes

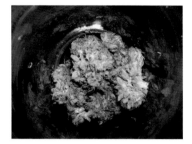

Strain: ACDC

Dominance: 50/50 (sativa dominant)
Parent Plants: Canatonic x Cannabis ruderalis
Grower: Resin Seeds
Awards: Numerous Cannabis Cup awards
THC: 1/20th of the CBD level
CBD: 19–56.9%
Flowering: Auto flowering
Yield: Up to 14 oz/m2 indoors; around the same per plant outdoors
Potential Positive Effects: Uplifting (H)
Potential Negative Effects: Dry Mouth (ExH)
Reported Treatment Uses: Pain (H), Stress (H), Anxiety (H), Epileptic Seizures (H), Cancer (H), MS (H)
Description: Smell is a pleasant sweet citrus with earthy undertones. Taste is a pleasant mix of sweet, peppery pine with an aftertaste of skunkiness.
Growing Hints: Bushy, up to 4 feet, needs support when it begins to bud. Likes minerals, especially magnesium and calcium.
Additional Notes: Very rare in that it is useful to patients suffering from a very wide array of diseases. Offers a whole-body relaxation, combined with mental focus. Fantastic medicinal strain that allows you to function fine mentally, since the THC is low. An extremely wide array of illnesses respond profoundly to ACDC. One woman who has ongoing pain from fibromyalgia wrote, "Thank God! After five puffs I was pain free for the first time in eighteen years." Great any time.

Notes

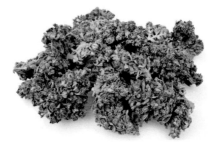

Strain: Afghani Bullrider
(a.k.a. Bull Rider)

Dominance: 100% indica
Parent Plants: Afggabu Kabdrace
Grower: West Coast Trading Co.
Awards: N/A
THC: 15–25%
CBD: 2%
Flowering: Not given, but outside matures in late October, early November
Yield: Has Good to High yields, whether indoors or outdoors
Potential Positive Effects: Relaxation (VH), Hungry (H), Euphoria (H)
Potential Negative Effects: Dry Mouth (VH), Anxiety (M), Paranoia (L), Dry Eyes (VL)
Reported Treatment Uses: Stress (VH), Pain (H), Insomnia (H), Muscle Spasms (MH), Depression (M)
Description: A beautiful, relatively short plant.
Growing Hints: Likes a Mediterranean climate, but should do well in heat.
Additional Notes: Developed by a Bull Rider in San Diego (specifically, Ocean Beach).

Notes

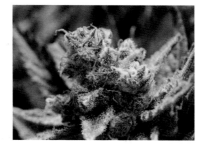

Strain: African

Dominance: 100% sativa (Landrace, Africa)
Parent Plants: Landrace
Grower: Unknown
Awards: N/A
THC: Not listed, but very strong
CBD: Not reported
Flowering: Typical sativa, so likely 11 weeks or more
Yield: Not reported
Potential Positive Effects: Euphoria (H), Happiness (H)
Potential Negative Effects: Dry Eyes (M)
Reported Treatment Uses: AIDS (H), Increased Energy (H), Depression (H), Appetite (H)
Description: Very strong. Various landrace crosses in Africa. Excellent reputation.
Growing Hints: None have been published but, as a sativa, you can expect it to be tall.
Additional Notes: Note lack of negative side effects. However, it is very strong!

Notes

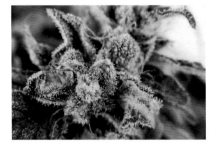

_____
_____
_____
_____
_____
_____
_____
_____
_____
_____
_____
_____
_____
_____
_____
_____
_____
_____
_____
_____

Strain: AK-47

Dominance: 65/35 (sativa dominant)
Parent Plants: Columbian x Mexican x Thai x Afghani
Grower: Serious Seeds
Awards: Winner of no less than 16 awards, including: Barcelona High Life Cup winner (hash, 2005); Toronto Treating Yourself Expo winner (sativa, 2011); *High Times* Cannabis Cup, third place (hybrid, 2011)
THC: 13–20%
CBD: 1%
Flowering: 8 to 9 weeks
Yield: High
Potential Positive Effects: Happiness (H), Euphoria (H), Uplifting (H), Relaxation (MH), Creativity (MH)
Potential Negative Effects: Dry Mouth (H), Dry Eyes (M), Dizziness (L), Paranoia (L), Headache (ExL)
Reported Treatment Uses: Stress (H), Anxiety (MH), Pain (MH), Depression (M), Insomnia (ML)
Description: Smell is sour and earthy. Taste has a hint of sweet flowers.
Growing Hints: Easy grow indoors or out.
Additional Notes: Hits quickly and with power like the weapon after which it is named. However, most report a mellow feeling accompanied by mental focus and creativity.

100 Best Cannabis Strains

Notes

Strain: Alaskan Thunderfuck

(a.k.a. ATF, Matanuska Thunderfuck, Matanuska Tundra)

Dominance: Percent not available (sativa-dominant cross)

Parent Plants: (Unknown x No. Cal. x Russian ruderalis) x Unknown Afghani

Grower: Unk.

Awards: 2011 Cannabis Cup winner (2011); *Rolling Stone* Best 5 Strains of 2017

THC: 16–23%

CBD: Not reported

Flowering: 12 weeks

Yield: 350g/m2 indoors. Outdoors depends on cultivation practices

Potential Positive Effects: Uplifting, Relaxation

Potential Negative Effects: Dry Mouth (H), Dry Eyes (M), Dizziness (VL), Paranoia (VL), Anxiety (VL)

Reported Treatment Uses: PTSD (H), Chronic Pain (H), Increased Energy (M)

Description: Very strong smell—like pine, menthol, lemon, and skunk. Tastes like banana and orange with a spicy chocolate aftertaste.

Growing Hints: Very easy grow but requires space and support of colas. Prone to mold and mildew.

Additional Notes: Clear-headed, creative, and productive.

Notes

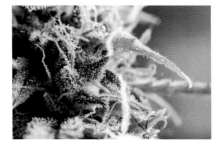

Strain: Amnesia Haze

Dominance: 80/20 (sativa dominant)
Parent Plants: South Asian Landrace x Jamaican Landrace
Grower: Difficult to find in US, extremely popular in Amsterdam
Awards: Cannabis Cup winner (sativa, 2004); Cannabis Cup winner (2012)
THC: 20–22%
CBD: 1%
Flowering: 12 weeks
Yield: 650g/m2 indoors; 700g/plant outdoors
Potential Positive Effects: Relaxation, but not sleepiness (H), Happiness (H)
Potential Negative Effects: Dry Mouth (M), Dry Eyes (M), Dizziness (L), Paranoia (VL), Headache (VL)
Reported Treatment Uses: PTSD (H), Autism (H), ADHD (H), Migraines (H)
Description: Has the taste of earthy lemony citrus and smells earthy and peppery.
Growing Hints: None published.
Additional Notes: Very popular strain.

100 Best Cannabis Strains

Notes

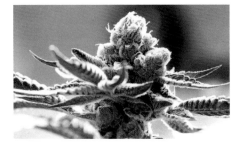

Strain: Apollo 13

Dominance: 85/15 (sativa dominant)
Parent Plants: P75 x Genius
Grower: Brothers Grimm
Awards: N/A
THC: 9%
CBD: Not reported
Flowering: 7 to 8 weeks
Yield: Heavy
Potential Positive Effects: Uplifting, Motivation, Happiness
Potential Negative Effects: Headache (H), Dry Mouth (M), Dry Eyes (L), Dizziness (L), Paranoia (L)
Reported Treatment Uses: Social Anxiety (H), Depression (H), Stress (H), Pain (H), Motivation (H), Creativity (H), Increased Energy (M)
Description: Tastes like herbal tea and skunk.
Growing Hints: Easy to grow, even for beginners.
Additional Notes: Hard to find but easy to grow for first timers. Moderate THC good for first-time users. Drinking lots of water is recommended.

100 Best Cannabis Strains

Notes

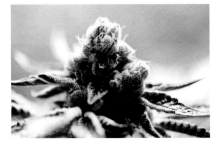

Strain: Aurora Indica

Dominance: 90/10 (indica dominant)
Parent Plants: Northern Lights x Afghani
Grower: Nirvana Seeds
Awards: None listed
THC: 14–19%
CBD: 0.1%
Flowering: 9 to 11 weeks
Yield: 10 to 14 oz/m2 indoors; 14 oz/plant outdoors
Potential Positive Effects: Relaxation (ExH),
    Sleepiness (H), Happiness (MH), Euphoria (MH), Uplifting (L)
Potential Negative Effects: Dry Mouth (ExH),
    Dry Eyes (L), Paranoia (VL)
Reported Treatment Uses: Pain (ExH), Stress (ExH),
    Insomnia (H), Muscle Spasms (MH), Depression (MH),
    ADHD (H)
Description: Smells like sweet earthy mango with a bit of
    lavender. Tastes like earthy, spicy mango with a sweet
    exhale.
Growing Hints: None available.
Additional Notes: Even though the THC levels are not
    super high, it is a powerful smoke. Couchlock is common
    with this strain.

100 Best Cannabis Strains

Notes

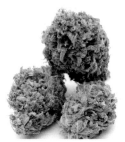

_____
_____
_____
_____
_____
_____
_____
_____
_____
_____
_____
_____
_____
_____
_____
_____
_____
_____
_____
_____
_____

Strain: Auto Critical Orange Punch

Dominance: 70/30 (indica dominant)
Parent Plants: Kritical Bilbo XXL (auto flowering—ruderalis) x Orange Punch
Grower: Dutch Passion
Awards: *High Times* Top 10 Strains of 2018
THC: Medium to Potent
CBD: Not reported
Flowering: 10 to 11 weeks
Yield: 450g/m2 indoors; outdoors 90g/plant
Potential Positive Effects: Euphoria, Happiness, Peaceful, Mental Clarity
Potential Negative Effects: Not given
Reported Treatment Uses: Stress (H)
Description: Tastes and smells like hashish, skunk, and citrus.
Growing Hints: 2 to 3 feet high, auto flowering. Does well indoors or outdoors, in almost any climate. Colas may need support. Give plenty of room for roots. Easy grow.
Additional Notes: Extremely popular. Balances a relaxed body and clear mind. Good day or night.

Notes

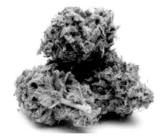

Strain: Bangi Haze

Dominance: 70/30 (sativa dominant)
Parent Plants: F8 stabilized Congolese x Nepalese Landraces
Grower: Ace Seeds
Awards: N/A
THC: 10–15%
CBD: 0.25%
Flowering: 11 weeks
Yield: 21oz/m2 indoors; 40oz/plant outdoors
Potential Positive Effects: Energetic (H), Hungry (H), Focused (H), Euphoria (L to H)
Potential Negative Effects: Dry Mouth (H), Dry Eyes (L), Paranoia (M)
Reported Treatment Uses: Stress (M), Pain (ML), Depression (VH), Insomnia (ML)
Description: Smells very sweet as well, with earthy berries, pungent herbal spices, and cheese. Tastes like berries and bananas with a hint of honey and cheese.
Growing Hints: Strongly resistant to both cold and mold. Likes a sunny, dry climate.
Additional Notes: When growing, the flower smells like floral lemon and anise.

Notes

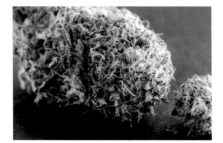

Strain: BC Big Bud

Dominance: 65/35 (sativa dominant)
Parent Plants: Big Bud x Unknown sativa strains
Grower: Parent plants vary among breeders
Awards: N/A
THC: 12–16%
CBD: 0.18–0.51%
Flowering: 8 to 9 weeks
Yield: Huge and Colossal have been terms used for this strain. Noted for giant buds and huge yields
Potential Positive Effects: Relaxation (M), Mellow (M)
Potential Negative Effects: Dry Mouth (M), Dry Eyes (M-L), Dizziness (L), Paranoia (VL), Anxiety (VL)
Reported Treatment Uses: Stress (H), Pain (MH), Depression (MH), Appetite (MH), Insomnia (MH)
Description: Noted for pressure field around eyes and forehead when effects first hit. Smells like skunky earth. Tastes like earth and sweet berries.
Growing Hints: Support for massive buds is essential.
Additional Notes: A true day or night strain.

100 Best Cannabis Strains

Notes

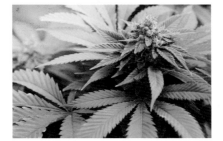

_____
_____
_____
_____
_____
_____
_____
_____
_____
_____
_____
_____
_____
_____
_____
_____
_____
_____
_____

Strain: Black Widow
(a.k.a. White Widow)

NOTE: *This is in reference to the origins of the strain, as opposed to what most now call White Widow.*

Dominance: 70/30 (indica dominant)

Parent Plants: Brazilian Landrace sativa x South India Landrace indica (three different phenotypes)

Grower: Developed by Shantibaba when co-owner of Green House Seeds—now Mr. Nice

Awards: Cannabis Cup winner (best indica, 1995)

THC: 24%

CBD: Not reported

Flowering: 8 to 10 weeks

Yield: 350 to 450g/m2 indoors; 300 to 400g/plant outdoors

Potential Positive Effects: Euphoria (MH), Happiness (MH), Relaxation (MH), Hungry (ML)

Potential Negative Effects: Dry Mouth (ML), Dry Eyes (ML), Dizziness (L), Paranoia, Headache (VL)

Reported Treatment Uses: Stress (M), Pain (M), Depression (ML), Insomnia (ML)

Description: Varies among the three different phenotypes.

Growing Hints: Considered difficult to grow.

Additional Notes: Hits hard and is long lasting.

Notes

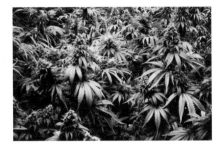

Strain: Blackberry

Dominance: 50/50 hybrid cross
Parent Plants: Black Domina x Raspberry Cough
Grower: Nirvana Seeds
Awards: N/A
THC: 20–26%
CBD: <1%
Flowering: 9 to 11 weeks
Yield: Reported only as High
Potential Positive Effects: Relaxation (M), Happiness (M), Euphoria (M), Sleepiness (ML), Uplifting (ML)
Potential Negative Effects: Dry Mouth (ML), Dry Eyes (ML), Dizziness (VL), Paranoia (VL), Headache (ExL)
Reported Treatment Uses: Pain (M), Stress (M), Anxiety (M), Insomnia (ML), Depression (ML)
Description: Has a profoundly pungent smell during growth. Taste is fruity and earthy.
Growing Hints: Requires strong ventilation and filtering when grown indoors, due to smell.
Additional Notes: Very strong. Small dosage recommended.

100 Best Cannabis Strains

Notes

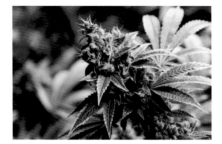

Strain: Blue Bastard

Dominance: 70/30 (indica dominant)
Parent Plants: DJ Short Blueberry x God Bud x White Widow
Grower: Unk
Awards: N/A
THC: 18–23%
CBD: 0%
Flowering: Not reported
Yield: High
Potential Positive Effects: Euphoria (ExH), Happiness (ExH)
Potential Negative Effects: Dry Mouth (M), Dry Eyes (M), Dizziness (M), Paranoia (M), Headache (M)
Reported Treatment Uses: Insomnia (H), Pain (MH), Stress (ExH), Arthritis (L), Alzheimer's (MH)
Description: Smells and tastes like pungent blueberries with the flavor of pine on the exhale.
Growing Hints: Not reported.
Additional Notes: "Hits like a truck . . . melt into whatever you are sitting on." Totally relaxed yet sociable/talkative and can be mobile. Giggles.

Notes

Strain: Blue Dragon

Dominance: 60/40 (indica dominant)
Parent Plants: Blueberry x Sour Diesel
Grower: Origins shrouded in secrecy, but feminized seeds can be purchased from Pacific Seed Bank
Awards: N/A
THC: Up to over 24%
CBD: 1%
Flowering: 8 to 10 weeks
Yield: 1 lb/m2 indoors; up to 19 oz/plant outdoors
Potential Positive Effects: Euphoria (VH), Happiness (VH), Relaxation (VH), Hungry (L)
Potential Negative Effects: Dry Mouth (ExH), Dry Eyes (M), Dizziness (VL), Paranoia (VL), Anxiety (ExL)
Reported Treatment Uses: Stress (ExH), Pain (VH), Insomnia (H), Appetite (M), Headaches (M)
Description: Tastes and smells like fuel and sweet berries.
Growing Hints: Resistant to powdery mildew and common diseases. Tall plant.
Additional Notes: Increasing in popularity due to medicinal effects. Very infrequent negative effects. Very balanced in indica/sativa effects.

Notes

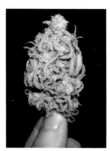

Strain: Blue Dream

Dominance: 60/40 (sativa dominant)

Note: Some list as a 80/20 sativa dominant, crossed with Blueberry x Silver Haze that has slightly lower THC and very little CBD

Parent Plants: Blueberry x Haze

Grower: Dark Heart Nursery

Awards: BDS Analytics lists as "The Most Popular Marijuana Strain"

THC: 17–24%

CBD: 2%

Flowering: 9 to 10 weeks

Yield: 21 oz/m2 indoors; up to 2 lb/plant outdoors

Potential Positive Effects: Euphoria (H), Happiness (H), Relaxation (H), Creativity (M)

Potential Negative Effects: Dry Mouth (ML), Dry Eyes (ML), Paranoia (L), Dizziness (L), Anxiety (VL)

Reported Treatment Uses: Stress (M), Anxiety (M), Depression (M), Nausea (M), Pain (M–L), Insomnia (L)

Description: Smells and tastes like sweet, fresh blueberries.

Growing Hints: Hearty, easy to grow plant with high yield but vulnerable to spider mites.

Additional Notes: Full body relaxation and cerebral invigoration. Easy grow, widespread availability.

Notes

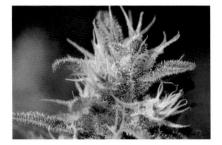

Strain: Blue Rhino

Dominance: 55/45 (indica dominant)
Parent Plants: Blueberry x White Rhino
Grower: DJ Short
Awards: N/A
THC: 15–20%
CBD: 2%
Flowering: 8 to 8.5 weeks
Yield: 500 to 600g/m2 indoors; 500g/plant outdoors
Potential Positive Effects: Euphoria (ExH), Relaxation (VH), Sleepiness (H), Uplifting (M)
Potential Negative Effects: Dry Mouth (ExH), Dry Eyes (H), Headache (VL), Dizziness (VL), Anxiety (VL)
Reported Treatment Uses: Pain (ExH), Stress (ExH), Muscle Spasms (VH), Depression (H), Insomnia (H)
Description: Tastes and smells like a combination of earthy and sweet with a skunky hint to the smell.
Growing Hints: Not reported.
Additional Notes: Very balanced between a head and body high. Relaxed, but also focused.

Notes

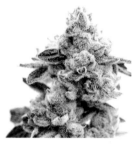

_____

_____

_____

_____

_____

_____

_____

_____

_____

_____

_____

_____

_____

_____

_____

_____

_____

_____

_____

_____

_____

Strain: Blue Zkittlez

Dominance: 70/30 (indica dominant)
Parent Plants: Blue Diamond x Zkittlez
Grower: Dying Breed Seeds
Awards: N/A
THC: 20%
CBD: 1%
Flowering: 8 to 9 weeks
Yield: Medium
Potential Positive Effects: Euphoria (M), Happiness (MH), Sleepiness (M), Relaxation (VH), Hungry (M)
Potential Negative Effects: Dry Mouth (H), Dry Eyes (VH), Dizziness (VL), Headache (VL), Anxiety (VL)
Reported Treatment Uses: Stress (VH), Pain (VH), Depression (H), Inflammation (M), Headaches (M), Appetite (M)
Description: Smells and tastes strongly of tart citrus, earth, berries, and wildflowers.
Growing Hints: Not difficult to grow, of medium height.
Additional Notes: Starts with a buzzing, which rapidly turns into an "insanely relaxed" state and at times causes sexual arousal.

Notes

Strain: Brainstorm Haze

Dominance: 90/10 (sativa dominant)
Parent Plants: Thai Landrace x Stargazer
Grower: Delta 9 Labs
Awards: N/A
THC: 14%
CBD: 0.1%
Flowering: 10 to 12 weeks
Yield: 500g to 600g/m2 indoors; varies/plant outdoors, but high yield
Potential Positive Effects: Creativity (M), Increased Energy (M)
Potential Negative Effects: Anxiety (VL), Dizziness (VL)
Reported Treatment Uses: Fatigue (H), Depression (H), Stress (M), Inflammation (M), Pain (VH)
Description: Tastes and smells fruity, floral, and spicy with earthy/skunky undertones.
Growing Hints: Loves SOG setup. Plants are short.
Additional Notes: There is another strain using this name that is made of the following: (Thai Haze x Sensi Star x Warlock) x AK-47. A sense of floating on air, with nothing being able to bring you down.

100 Best Cannabis Strains

Notes

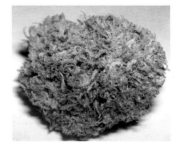

Strain: Bubba Kush

Dominance: Indica dominant
Parent Plants: Bubble Gum x Kush
Grower: Green House Seeds
Awards: N/A
THC: 27%
CBD: Not reported
Flowering: 9 weeks
Yield: Different sources describe the yield as Sizable and Excellent
Potential Positive Effects: Relaxation (VH), Sleepiness (H), Euphoria (H), Hungry (MH)
Potential Negative Effects: Dry Mouth (H), Dry Eyes (ML), Dizzy (L), Paranoia (VL), Headache (ExL)
Reported Treatment Uses: Stress (VH), Pain (H), Insomnia (H), Anxiety (MH), Depression (M), PTSD (H), Nerve Pain (VH), Sleep Apnea (H), Arthritis (H), ADHD (H)
Description: Smells like extremely sweet hash and pine. Tastes like sweet hashish with a hint of chocolate and coffee on the exhale.
Growing Hints: Thrives in both a SOG and SCROG setup.
Additional Notes: Exceptionally strong. Start VERY slow with this one.
Note: There is now a strain called "Bubby Kush CBD" that is only 8% THC and 10% CBD.

Notes

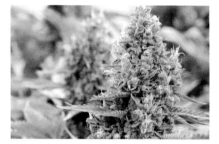

Strain: Bubba OG

Dominance: 80/20 (indica dominant)
Parent Plants: Bubba Kush (pre-1998) x Ghost OG
Grower: Dr. Greenthumb Seeds
Awards: N/A
THC: 22–25%
CBD: 8–10%
Flowering: 9 to 10 weeks
Yield: 350 to 450/m2 in SOG or SCROG setup indoors, 900g/
plant outdoors
Potential Positive Effects: Relaxed (HM), Happy (M),
Sleepiness (M), Euphoric (M), Appetite (M)
Potential Negative Effects: Dry Mouth (L), Dry Eyes
(VL), Dizziness (ExL), Paranoia (ExL), Headache (ExL)
Reported Treatment Uses: Stress (M), Pain (M), Insomnia
(M), Anxiety (M), Depression (L)
Description: Smells like sweet and pungent flowers. Tastes
like earthy hash and fruity diesel.
Growing Hints: 1.5 to 2 ft indoors; 3 to 10 ft outdoors;
indoors craves a SOG or SCROG setup.
Additional Notes: Flavor of Bubba, potency of OG, and a
better yield than either of them.

Notes

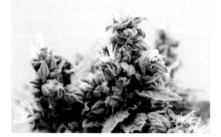

Strain: Bubblicious

Dominance: 70/30 (indica dominant). Note: Some list as 60/40
Parent Plants: Original Bubblegum x F1 Lavender
Grower: Nirvana Seeds
Awards: N/A
THC: 15–20%
CBD: Not reported
Flowering: 8 to 11 weeks
Yield: 400 to 500g/m2 indoors if grown with a SCROG setup; 1 lb/plant outdoors
Potential Positive Effects: Relaxation (ExH), Focused (MH), Talkative (M), Happiness (M), Creativity (LM)
Potential Negative Effects: Dry Mouth (ExH), Dry Eyes (L), Headache (ExL), Paranoia (ExL), Anxiety (ExL)
Reported Treatment Uses: Pain (ExH), Depression (ExH), Nausea (VH), Stress (VH), Cramps (HM)
Description: Smells like fruity, blueberry citrus bubblegum; tastes like fruity, earthy, skunky sweet bubblegum.
Growing Hints: Susceptible to mold. Likes Mediterranean climate.
Additional Notes: Many consider this the "best" strain due to taste, smell, very low side effects, and medicinal uses. Very relaxed, yet energized.

Notes

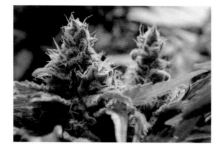

Strain: Buddha's Love

Dominance: 75/25 (sativa dominant)
Parent Plants: Original Bubblegum x F1 Lavender
Grower: Nirvana Seeds
Awards: N/A
THC: 15–20%
CBD: Not reported
Flowering: 8 to 11 weeks
Yield: 400g to 500g/m2 indoors; varies/plant outdoors
Potential Positive Effects: Sexual arousal
Potential Negative Effects: Dizziness (VL), Dry Eyes (VL)
Reported Treatment Uses: Pain (H), Stress (H),
    Appetite (H), Depression (H)
Description: Tastes and smells fruity, floral, and spicy with an
    earthy/skunky undertone.
Growing Hints: Loves SOG setup. Plants are short.
Additional Notes: Almost zero negative side effects. Many
    patients consider it the best medicinal strain available.

Notes

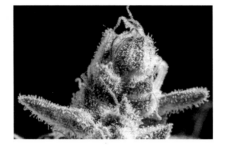

Strain: Buddha's Sister

Dominance: 80/20 (indica dominant)
Parent Plants: Reclining Buddha x Afghani-Hawaiian
Grower: Soma Seeds
Awards: *High Times* Cannabis Cup runner-up (indica)
THC: 19–22%
CBD: 0.1%
Flowering: 8 to 9 weeks
Yield: Differing sources say Pleasing or High
Potential Positive Effects: Relaxation (H), Euphoria (M), Uplifting (M), Sleepiness (M)
Potential Negative Effects: Dry Mouth (ML), Dry Eyes (L), Anxiety (VL), Dizziness (VL), Paranoia (VL)
Reported Treatment Uses: Stress (MH), Anxiety (MH), Pain (M), Insomnia (M), Depression (M)
Description: Smells like tart cherries; tastes like SweetTarts cherry candies.
Growing Hints: Grows lots of side limbs; easy to grow by any method. Mold resistant.
Additional Notes: Very powerful and should not be over smoked. High trichome level and great for making hash.

Notes

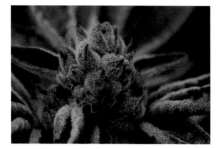

Strain: Butterscotch

Dominance: 50/50 (though totally indica effects)
Parent Plants: Unknown
Grower: Unknown
Awards: N/A
THC: 18.5–21%
CBD: 0.2%
Flowering: 8 to 9 weeks
Yield: 1 lb/m2 indoors; a little over 1 lb/plant outdoors
Potential Positive Effects: Relaxing
Potential Negative Effects: Dry Mouth (H), Dry Eyes (H), Dizziness (H)
Reported Treatment Uses: Stress (H), Insomnia (H), Relaxation (H), Shingles (H), Appetite (MH), Nausea (H), Inflammation (M), PMS (H), PTSD (H), Migraine (MH), Anxiety (MH)
Description: Said to have the best aroma of any strain— exactly like its name. Taste is nutty pine with citrus.
Growing Hints: Very easy to grow and resistant to almost all molds and diseases.
Additional Notes: Anxiety can appear with new users. Effects can calm both mind and body.

Notes

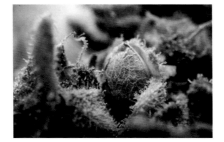

Strain: Canna Sutra

Dominance: 70/30 (indica dominant)
Parent Plants: Reclining Buddha x Sensi Star
Grower: Delta-9 Labs
Awards: N/A
THC: 13–17%
CBD: <1%
Flowering: 9 to 10 weeks
Yield: 11 to 18oz/m2 indoors; 11 or more oz/plant outdoors
Potential Positive Effects: Euphoria (ExH), Relaxation (ExH), Sleepiness (VH), Happiness (VH), Sexual Arousal (M)
Potential Negative Effects: Dry Mouth (VH)
Reported Treatment Uses: Pain (Ex H), Headaches (VH), Insomnia (M), Stress (M), Muscle Spasms (M)
Description: Smells like sweet berries, yet pungent and earthy. Tastes sweet, fruity berry, herbal, and earthy.
Growing Hints: Likes a warm climate.
Additional Notes: The most famous of the strains that promote sexual arousal and enhance sexual experience.

Notes

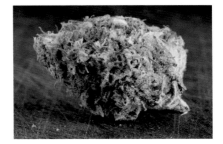

Strain: Casey Jones

Dominance: 80/20 (sativa dominant)
Parent Plants: Trainwreck x Sour Diesel
Grower: Devil's Harvest
Awards: N/A
THC: 22%
CBD: 0.2%
Flowering: 9 to 10 weeks
Yield: 14oz/m2 indoors; 17oz/plant outdoors
Potential Positive Effects: Energetic (H), Hungry (H), Focused (H), Euphoria (ML to MH)
Potential Negative Effects: Dry Mouth (H), Dry Eyes (L), Paranoia (M)
Reported Treatment Uses: Stress (M), Pain (ML), Depression (VH), Insomnia (ML)
Description: Smells lemony with a hint of bubble gum. Tastes like strong, sweet citrus. Earthy lemon when exhaled.
Growing Hints: Prefers Mediterranean climate.
Additional Notes: This is a strain that has been increasing in popularity every year since it was developed.

Notes

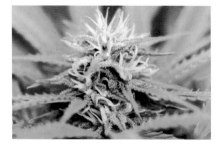

Strain: CBD Blue Shark

Dominance: 70/30 (indica dominant)
Parent Plants: CBD Shark x Blue Cheese
Grower: Barney's Farm
Awards: N/A
THC: 6.5%
CBD: 6.5%
Flowering: 8 to 9 weeks
Yield: 550g/m2 indoors; 550g/plant outdoors
Potential Positive Effects: Happiness (L), Focused (MH), Relaxation (VH), Hungry (MH)
Potential Negative Effects: Dizziness (VH), Dry Mouth (VL), Dry Eyes (VL), Headache (VL), Anxiety (VL)
Reported Treatment Uses: Stress (VH), Pain (VH), Depression (H), Inflammation (VH), Fatigue (H)
Description: Smells and tastes floral, jasmine, berry, and cheese.
Growing Hints: An "easy grow" strain. About 3.5 feet tall.
Additional Notes: Very balanced in THC and CBD. Despite high reports of dizziness, people report enjoying this strain very much.

Notes

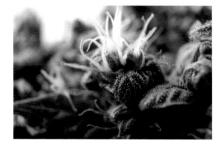

Strain: Charlotte's Web

Dominance: Ruderalis
Parent Plants: Breeders' Secret
Grower: Stanley Brothers
Awards: Widely recognized as the most dominant CBD strain available
THC: 0.3%
CBD: 42–47%—over 600 times as most recreational marijuana strains
Flowering: 8 to 9 weeks
Yield: High
Potential Positive Effects: Relaxation (ExH), Creativity (H), Sedated (ML), Focused (MH)
Potential Negative Effects: Dry Mouth (L), Dry Eyes (L), Dizziness (VL), Headache (ExL), Anxiety (ExL)
Reported Treatment Uses: Pain (ExH), Nausea (VH), Appetite (MH), Epileptic Seizures (ExH), Inflammation (ExH), Muscle Cramps (H), Migraines (M)
Description: Information on taste and smell not available.
Growing Hints: Clones only, and only from the Stanley Brothers.
Additional Notes: Legal in many states as "hemp" (0.3% THC or under) where marijuana is still illegal. NO high/stoned from this strain. Near 0% THC. Named after Charlotte Figi, who experienced reduced epileptic seizures (brought on by Dravet syndrome) from the strain, which is now used often to treat toddlers and children dealing with epilepsy.

Notes

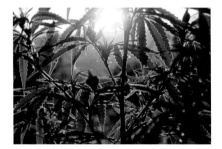

Strain: Cheese

Dominance: 60/40 (indica dominant)

Parent Plants: Skunk #1 x Afghani indica strain

Grower: Royal Queen Seeds/Big Huddha Seeds

Awards: World famous and highly praised for its taste and effects, yet no awards listed

THC: 14–20%

CBD: <1%

Flowering: 9 to 10 weeks

Yield: 14oz/m2 indoors; 21oz/plant outdoors

Potential Positive Effects: Relaxation (ExH), Euphoria (VH), Happiness (VH), Uplifting (MH), Hungry (M), Giggles (H)

Potential Negative Effects: Dry Mouth (MH), Dry Eyes (M–H), Paranoia (VL), Dizziness (VL), Headache (ExL)

Reported Treatment Uses: Stress (ExH), Pain (VH), Depression (MH), Insomnia (M), Appetite (M)

Description: Popular due to its unusual fragrant characteristics. Dubbed the "stinky socks" of strains, it smells and tastes exactly like ripe cheese: earthy, sweet, pungent, creamy, skunky, and woody.

Growing Hints: Loves a sunny, Mediterranean climate. Easy grow. Tall.

Additional Notes: One of the most popular strains for a very long time. Used in developing many other strains. Considered a "happy strain," good for both day and evening use.

Notes

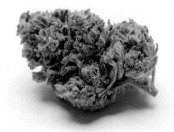

_____
_____
_____
_____
_____
_____
_____
_____
_____
_____
_____
_____
_____
_____
_____
_____
_____
_____
_____
_____
_____

Strain: Chem Scout

Dominance: 60/40 (indica dominant)
Parent Plants: Chemdawg 91 x Girl Scout Cookies (GSC)
Grower: IC Collective
Awards: *High Times* Cannabis Cup top honors (2014, San Francisco); *High Times* 10 Best Strains of 2018
THC: 20–26%
CBD: 0.2%
Flowering: 7 to 9 weeks
Yield: 10 to 14 oz/m2 indoors; 14 oz/plant outdoors
Potential Positive Effects: Relaxation (ExH), Euphoria (MH), Focused (M), Sleepiness (ML)
Potential Negative Effects: Dry Mouth (ExH), Dry Eyes (ExL), Dizziness (ExL), Paranoia (ExL), Anxiety (ExL)
Reported Treatment Uses: Stress (VH), Muscle Spasms (M), Depression (M), Pain (M), Fatigue (M)
Description: Smells earthy, skunky, citrusy, and like nutty coffee. Tastes sweet, citrusy, nutty, and piney.
Growing Hints: Mediterranean climate. Ready for harvest in late September or early October.
Additional Notes: Most consider it better than either of its highly acclaimed parent strains. Extremely potent.

Notes

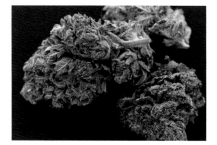

_____
_____
_____
_____
_____
_____
_____
_____
_____
_____
_____
_____
_____
_____
_____
_____
_____
_____
_____

Strain: Chernobyl

Dominance: 80/20 (sativa dominant)
Parent Plants: Trainwreck x Jack the Ripper x Trinity
Grower: Not reported
Awards: N/A
THC: 16–22%
CBD: 0.1%
Flowering: 8 to 9 weeks
Yield: 14oz/m2 indoors; 14oz/plant outdoors
Potential Positive Effects: Uplifting (VH), Relaxation (H), Happiness (VH), Euphoria (H), Energetic (H)
Potential Negative Effects: Dry Mouth (H), Dry Eyes (M), Paranoia (L), Anxiety (M), Dizziness (L)
Reported Treatment Uses: Stress (VH), Pain (H), Depression (VH), Nausea (M), Fatigue (M)
Description: Smells and tastes earthy, sweet and sour lemon with a hint of cherry.
Growing Hints: Tall plant that wants warm and sunny, but not hot. Highly resistant to diseases.
Additional Notes: "The ultimate happy smoke."

Notes

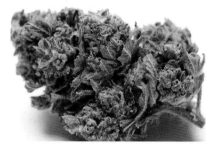

_____

_____

_____

_____

_____

_____

_____

_____

_____

_____

_____

_____

_____

_____

_____

_____

_____

_____

_____

Strain: Cherry Pie

Dominance: 80/20 (indica dominant)
Parent Plants: Grandaddy Purple x Durban Poison
Grower: Not reported
Awards: N/A
THC: 16–24%
CBD: 1%
Flowering: 8 to 9 weeks
Yield: 1 lb/m2 indoors; 1 lb/plant outdoors
Potential Positive Effects: Euphoria (MH), Uplifting (MH), Relaxing (H), Creativity (M)
Potential Negative Effects: Dry Mouth (M), Dry Eyes (M), Dizzy (VL), Anxiety (ExL), Paranoia (ExL)
Reported Treatment Uses: PTSD (H), Anxiety (M), Bipolar Disorder, Migraines (H), Stress (H), Muscle Stiffness (H), Insomnia (L), Depression (ML)
Description: Smells like cherry pie.
Growing Hints: Prefers 70- to 80-degree Mediterranean climate.
Additional Notes: Hard to find authentic, as many other combinations go by this name. Liked by newbies and old-time users alike. Worth getting the real thing.

100 Best Cannabis Strains

Notes

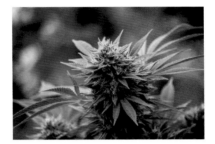

Strain: Chocolope

Dominance: 95/5 (sativa dominant)
Parent Plants: OG Chocolate Thai x Cannalope Haze
Grower: DNA Genetics
Awards: 1st Hydro Highlife Cup winner (sativa, 2008); 2 *High Times* Cannabis Cup runner-up (sativa, 2010); Coffeeshop *High Times* Cannabis Cup runner-up (sativa, 2007); Hydrolife Cup runner-up (sativa, 2007); Outdoor Spannabis runner-up (sativa, 2011); Hydro Highlife Cup, third place (sativa, 2009); Coffeeshop *High Times* Cannabis Cup, third place (sativa, 2008); Indoor 4th Edition Buenos Aires, Argentina, third place (sativa, 2011); Indoor Bio Spannabis, third place (sativa, 2008); Hollyweed Cup, third place (sativa, 2006); Strain of the Year (2007)
THC: 16–21%
CBD: 0.2%
Flowering: 8 to 9+ weeks (Exceptionally short flowering time for a sativa)
Yield: 500 to 600g/m2 indoors; 750 to 900g/plant outdoors
Potential Positive Effects: Creativity, Energetic
Potential Negative Effects: Dry Mouth (VH), Dry Eyes (H), Anxiety (VL), Paranoia (VL), Dizziness (VL), Headaches (VL)
Reported Treatment Uses: PTSD (H), Stress (VH), Fatigue (M), Pain (M), Appetite (L), Asthma (M)
Description: Tastes and smells like chocolate, coffee, and vanilla.
Growing Hints: Exceptionally easy to grow but requires outdoor space and support of colas. Prefers Mediterranean climate. Prone to mold and mildew.
Additional Notes: Clear-headed feelings of creativity and productiveness.

Notes

Strain: Chronic

Dominance: 50/50 hybrid cross
Parent Plants: Northern Lights x AK-47 x Skunk #1
Grower: Serious Seeds
Awards: *High Times* Cannabis Cup, third place (hybrid cross, 1994); numerous awards since
THC: 13–22%
CBD: 0.2–1.8%
Flowering: 8 to 9 weeks
Yield: 14 to 21 oz/m2 indoors; 25 or more oz/plant outdoors
Potential Positive Effects: Happiness (ExH), Talkative (VH), Energized (MH), Giggles (MH), Uplifting (MH)
Potential Negative Effects: Dry Mouth (ExH), Dry Eyes (ExL), Dizziness (ExL), Paranoia (ExL), Anxiety (ExL)
Reported Treatment Uses: Depression (ExH), Stress (VH), Pain (MH), Insomnia (M), Eye Pressure (M)
Description: Smells like honey, flowers, and spices.
Growing Hints: Likes a semi-humid climate—easy grow.
Additional Notes: Loyalists refer to this strain as a "living legend."

Notes

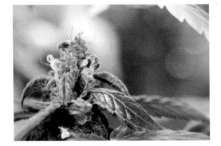

Strain: Confidential Cheese

Dominance: 55/45 (indica dominant)
Parent Plants: Cheese x LA Confidential
Grower: DNA Genetics
Awards: N/A
THC: 16%
CBD: 1%
Flowering: 8 to 9 weeks
Yield: 18oz/m2 indoors; 1 lb/plant outdoors
Potential Positive Effects: Relaxation (ExH), Happiness (MH), Sleepiness (M), Hungry (M), Uplifting (M)
Potential Negative Effects: Dry Mouth (VH), Dry Eyes (VH), Anxiety (VL), Dizziness (VL), Headache (VL)
Reported Treatment Uses: Stress (ExH), Pain (VH), Nausea (MH), Insomnia (M), Depression (M)
Description: No additional information available.
Growing Hints: Must continually remove leaves from flowering spikes for light and free air flow or disease will result. Prune heavily for good yield.
Additional Notes: Total relaxation with a completely clear and focused mind.

Notes

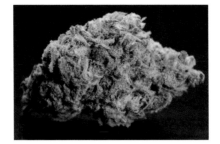

_____
_____
_____
_____
_____
_____
_____
_____
_____
_____
_____
_____
_____
_____
_____
_____
_____
_____
_____

Strain: Creme de la Creme

Dominance: 70/30 (indica dominant)
Parent Plants: Strawdawg Illuminati Cut x Chemdogging
Grower: Mephisto Genetics
Awards: N/A
THC: 20+%
CBD: 0.5%
Flowering: 9 to 10 weeks
Yield: 400g/m2
Potential Positive Effects: Relaxation
Potential Negative Effects: Couchlock (VH)
Reported Treatment Uses: Aches and Pains (VH),
Insomnia (VH)
Description: Tastes and smells pungent. Intense chemical
smell and taste with a flowery tone.
Growing Hints: Prefers an 11–13 hour light cycle for indoor
grows. Only 1.5 to 2.5 ft tall.
Additional Notes: An F-4 hybrid. Potent with long-lasting
effects.

Notes

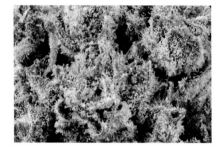

Strain: Critical Mass

Dominance: 60/40 (sativa dominant)
Parent Plants: Skunk #1 x Afghani
Grower: Mr. Nice Seed Bank
Awards: N/A
THC: 19–22%
CBD: 5%
Flowering: 6 to 8 weeks
Yield: Huge: 27oz/m2indoors; up to 6 lb/plant outdoors
Potential Positive Effects: Relaxation (VH), Euphoria (H), Sleepiness (MH), Uplifting (M)
Potential Negative Effects: Dry Mouth (M), Dry Eyes (L), Dizzy (VL), Anxiety (VL), Paranoia (VL)
Reported Treatment Uses: Pain (H), Stress (H), Anxiety (MH), Depression (M), Insomnia (M)
Description: Mild smell (though pungent in growing stage). Tastes both sweet and earthy.
Growing Hints: Susceptible to mold—use organic spray—otherwise an easy grow. Support needed. Mediterranean climate or indoors to discourage mold.
Additional Notes: Grows up to 10 feet; requires support or will break.

100 Best Cannabis Strains

Notes

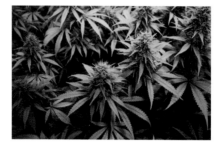

Strain: Darth Vader OG

Dominance: 100% indica cross
Parent Plants: Afghani x Kush
Grower: Blue Hemp
Awards: N/A
THC: 12–14%
CBD: 1%
Flowering: 8 to 9 weeks
Yield: Average
Potential Positive Effects: Sleepiness (ExH), Relaxation (VH), Euphoria (MH), Happiness (MH), Hungry (M)
Potential Negative Effects: Dry Mouth (VH), Dry Eyes (VH), Headache (ExL), Paranoia (ExL), Dizziness (ExL)
Reported Treatment Uses: Insomnia (ExH), Stress (VH), Pain (M), Inflammation (M), Depression (LM)
Description: Smells sweet, spicy, floral, earthy, and peppery. Taste is a subtle skunky grape.
Growing Hints: Very dark, short plant that does not branch much and can flourish without additional supports.
Additional Notes: No additional notes reported.

Notes

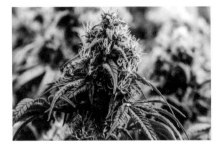

_____

_____

_____

_____

_____

_____

_____

_____

_____

_____

_____

_____

_____

_____

_____

_____

_____

_____

_____

_____

_____

Strain: Durban Poison

Dominance: 100% sativa landrace
Parent Plants: Landrace sativa from South African port city of Durban
Grower: Landrace
Awards: Top 3 bestselling strains in Colorado, 2015
THC: 10–24%
CBD: 0.2%
Flowering: 9 to 10 weeks (very short flowering time for a sativa)
Yield: 13oz/m2 indoors; 1 LB+/plant outdoors
Potential Positive Effects: Uplifting, Energetic, Happiness, Euphoria, Creativity, Focus
Potential Negative Effects: Dry Mouth (VH), Dry Eyes (M), Anxiety (L), Paranoia (L), Headaches (VL)
Reported Treatment Uses: ADHD (H), Appetite Suppressant (H), Stress (VH), Depression (VH), Pain (M), Fatigue (M), Nausea (L)
Description: Tastes and smells earthy, piney, spicy, and herbal.
Growing Hints: Easy to grow but very tall. Resistant to both mold and pests.
Additional Notes: Very popular since brought to the US in the 1970s by Ed Rosenthal.

Notes

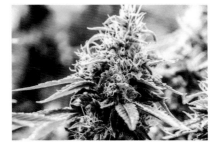

_____
_____
_____
_____
_____
_____
_____
_____
_____
_____
_____
_____
_____
_____
_____
_____
_____
_____
_____

Strain: Forbidden Fruit
(a.k.a. Le Fruit Defendu)

Dominance: 70/30 (indica dominant)
Parent Plants: Cherry Pie x Tangie
Grower: Multiple breeders
Awards: N/A
THC: 23–26%
CBD: 0.2%
Flowering: Not reported
Yield: Not reported
Potential Positive Effects: Euphoria (M), Happiness (MH), Sleepiness (M), Relaxation (VH)
Potential Negative Effects: Dry Mouth (VH), Dry Eyes (M), Paranoia (VL), Dizziness (VL), Anxiety (VL)
Reported Treatment Uses: Stress (VH), Pain (H), Depression (H), Insomnia (MH), Muscle Spasms (M)
Description: Dense buds, deep purple hues, dark green leaves, and wiry orange hairs. Considered to be the strongest (and best) smelling pot *ever*; smelling and tasting of cherries, mangos, pine, and passion fruit candy.
Growing Hints: Most seeds are auto blooming requiring a 12hr/12hr light cycle.
Additional Notes: People are wild about this strain, and while it has medicinal value you will experience couchlock; it is very strong and should be used *with moderation*. Failure to do so can result in anxiety. It is one of those strains . . . while a little is outstanding, a lot is *not* good at all.

Notes

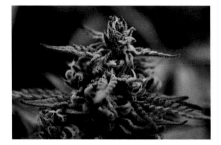

Strain: French Cookies

Dominance: 60/40 (sativa dominant)
Parent Plants: Platinum Cookies phenotype
Grower: TH Seeds
Awards: *High Times* Top 10 Strains of 2018
THC: 15–23%
CBD: 1%
Flowering: 9 to 10 weeks
Yield: About 1 lb/m2 indoors; 1 lb/plant outdoors
Potential Positive Effects: Uplifting, Energetic, Clarity, Focus
Potential Negative Effects: None listed
Reported Treatment Uses: New strain—incomplete, but said to be "ideal" for treating Fatigue, Depression, Stress, ADHD, Migraines, and Headaches.
Description: Smells like grapes and fruitiness. Tastes like grapes and cookies.
Growing Hints: Grows to about 4 feet. Purple and blue leaves and a covering of sticky trichomes.
Additional Notes: A light boost that is anxiety-free.

Notes

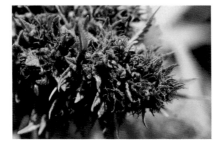

Strain: G 13 Haze

Dominance: 82/20 (sativa dominant)

Parent Plants: G13 x Haze

Grower: Origin unknown—Barney's Farm offers a G13/ Hawaiian Haze of this name

Awards: N/A

THC: 22–24%

CBD: 0.25%

Flowering: 11 weeks

Yield: 21oz/m2 indoors; 40oz/plant outdoors

Potential Positive Effects: Relaxation (H), Euphoria (MH), Happiness (MH), Sleepiness (M)

Potential Negative Effects: Dry Mouth (H), Dry Eyes (L), Dizziness (L), Paranoia (L), Headache (VL)

Reported Treatment Uses: Stress (VH), Pain (MH), Depression (MH), Insomnia (M), Headache (M–L)

Description: Smells berry, earthy, pungent, skunky, and sweet. Tastes sweet, woody, and piney.

Growing Hints: Not particularly tall for a typical sativa. High resistance to disease.

Additional Notes: A great deal of rumor about the origin, including that it was "designed" by the government.

Notes

Strain: Ghost Train Haze

Dominance: 80/20 (sativa dominant)
Parent Plants: Ghost OG x Nevil's Wreck
Grower: Kyle Kushman
Awards: #1 Best Colorado Sativa Flower (Denver, 2015)
THC: 27%
CBD: 0.2%
Flowering: 9 to 11 weeks
Yield: 10oz/m2 indoors; 14oz/plant outdoors
Potential Positive Effects: Uplifting (VH), Happiness (VH), Euphoria (VH), Energized (H) Focused (MH)
Potential Negative Effects: Dry Mouth (M), Dry Eyes (M), Paranoia (M), Anxiety (H), Dizziness (L)
Reported Treatment Uses: Stress (VH), Pain (MH), Depression (VH), Inflammation (M), Fatigue (M)
Description: Smells earthy citrus, floral, pungent and tastes earthy, citrus, and sweet lemon.
Growing Hints: Wants hot and dry (Mediterranean) climate.
Additional Notes: A very pleasant experience for most.

Notes

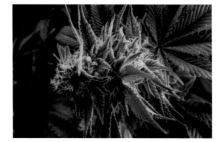

Strain: Girl Scout Cookies
(a.k.a. GSC)

Dominance: 60/40 (indica dominant)
Parent Plants: OG Kush x Durban Poison x Cherry Kush
Grower: Unknown breeder, but originated in San Francisco Bay Area
Awards: Multiple Cannabis Cup Awards
THC: 19–28%
CBD: 1%
Flowering: 9 to 10 weeks
Yield: 10 oz/m2 or /plant
Potential Positive Effects: Euphoria (H), Relaxation (H), Uplifting (H), Creativity (M)
Potential Negative Effects: Dry Mouth (M), Dry Eyes (L), Dizzy (ExL), Paranoia (ExL), Anxiety (ExL)
Reported Treatment Uses: Stress (H), Depression (M), Pain (M), Anxiety (M), Insomnia (ML), PTSD, Appetite
Description: Smells and tastes sweet and earthy.
Growing Hints: Strongly resistant to both mildew and pests. Loves a SG setup.
Additional Notes: Girl Scouts of America recently successfully sued in Oregon to prevent dispensaries from using the name, and it is now referred to as "GSC."

Notes

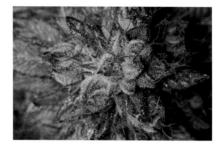

Strain: GMO Cookies
(a.k.a. Garlic Cookies)

Dominance: 90/10 (indica dominant)
Parent Plants: Chemdog x Girl Scout Cookies (GSC)
Grower: Mamiko Seeds
Awards: N/A
THC: 20–24%
CBD: Not reported
Flowering: 10 weeks
Yield: 1 LB/m2 indoors; outdoors, 600g/plant (1.3 LBs)
Potential Positive Effects: Relaxation (ExH), Happiness (H), Euphoria (M)
Potential Negative Effects: Dry Mouth (ExH), Dry Eyes (L), Insomnia (MH), Headaches (ML), Anxiety (ML), Dizziness (L)
Reported Treatment Uses: Depression (VH), Pain (MH), Stress (MH), Anxiety (M), Appetite Suppressant (M)
Description: Smells like pungent, spicy coffee. Tastes like delicious savory garlic with a pungent exhale.
Growing Hints: Not reported.
Additional Notes: Extremely unusual for a strain to *decrease* appetite. Also, unusual for an indica-dominant strain to fail to result in sleepiness.

100 Best Cannabis Strains

Notes

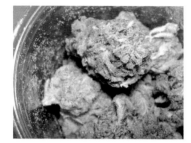

Strain: God's Gift

Dominance: 90/10 (indica dominant)
Parent Plants: Granddaddy Purple x OG Kush
Grower: Multiple growers
Awards: Best Indica Biocup (Spain, 2015)
THC: 18–27%
CBD: 1%
Flowering: 8 to 9 weeks
Yield: 10oz/m2 indoors; 10oz/plant outdoors
Potential Positive Effects: Uplifting (M), Happiness (H), Relaxation (VH), Euphoria (M), Sleepiness (M), Giggles (M)
Potential Negative Effects: Dry Mouth (VH), Dry Eyes (M), Paranoia (VL), Headache (VL), Dizziness (VL)
Reported Treatment Uses: Stress (VH), Pain (H), Depression (H), Insomnia (M), Anxiety (M)
Description: Smells earthy grape, spicy sweet. Tastes like berry, citrus, grape, woody, and sweet.
Growing Hints: This is a short, easy to grow plant with a high resistance to diseases.
Additional Notes: Demand was so high from 2004 through 2006 that dispensaries could not keep up with the demand and constantly ran out of stock.

Notes

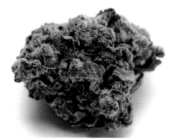

Strain: Gorilla Glue #4

Dominance: 50/50 hybrid cross
Parent Plants: Chem's Sister x Sound Dubb x Chocolate Diesel
Grower: Developed by Joesy Whales of GG Strains
Awards: Multiple Cannabis Cups in 2014, as well as the
   Jamaican World Cup
THC: 25–30%
CBD: 0.1%
Flowering: 8 to 9 weeks
Yield: 18 oz/m2 indoors; 21 oz/plant outdoors
Potential Positive Effects: Relaxation (ExH), Euphoria
   (H), Happiness (H), Uplifting (M), Sleepiness (ML)
Potential Negative Effects: Dry Mouth (ExH), Dry Eyes (M),
   Paranoia (ML), Anxiety (VL), Headache (VL), Couchlock (H)[1]
Reported Treatment Uses: Stress (ExH), Depression (H),
   Pain (H), Insomnia (M), Appetite (M)
Description: Smells like pine, spices, sandalwood, sweet cher-
   ries, and berries. Tastes earthy, pungent, piney, diesel, coffee,
   and like chemicals.
Growing Hints: Likes it sunny and warm. Highly resistant to
   disease. Easy grow.
Additional Notes: Gorilla Glue #4 got its name from
   the fact that growers had a hard time trimming its buds,
   with the high resin content leading their scissors to stick
   together.

---

1 Some do not consider couchlock as a "negative"—especially for those
   who otherwise have a lot of pain.

100 Best Cannabis Strains

Notes

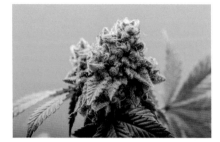

Strain: Granddaddy Purple

Dominance: 80/20 (indica dominant)
Parent Plants: Purple Urkle x Big Bud
Grower: Den Estes
Awards: *High Times* Medical Cannabis Cup, Highest CBD
    Trophy (Los Angeles, 2015). Has a long history as a breeding
    parent of award-winning offspring
THC: 17–27%
CBD: 7%
Flowering: 8 to 9 weeks
Yield: 15g to 95g/plant indoors; 225g to 2,250g/plant outdoors
Potential Positive Effects: Relaxation (VH), Hungry (M),
    Euphoria (MH), Sleepiness (MH), Happiness (MH)
Potential Negative Effects: Dry Mouth (VH), Anxiety (L),
    Paranoia (L), Dry Eyes (M), Dizzy (L)
Reported Treatment Uses: Stress (VH), Pain (VH),
    Insomnia (VH), Appetite (M), Depression (MH)
Description: Very rare to have high CBD with high THC.
    Beautiful purple plant.
Growing Hints: Easy grow indoors and out.
Additional Notes: *The* most popular medicinal strain to
    date.

Notes

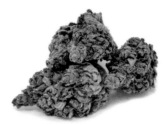

_____
_____
_____
_____
_____
_____
_____
_____
_____
_____
_____
_____
_____
_____
_____
_____
_____
_____

Strain: Grape Ape

Dominance: 90/10 (indica dominant)
Parent Plants: Mendocino Purps x Skunk x Afghani
Grower: Apothecary Genetics and Barney's Farm
Awards: Cannabis Cup winner (best wax, 2011)
THC: 18–21%
CBD: 0%
Flowering: 7 to 8 weeks
Yield: 16 oz/m2 indoors; 28 oz/plant outdoors
Potential Positive Effects: Relaxation (VH), Hungry (M),
    Euphoria (M), Sleepiness (MH), Happiness (MH)
Potential Negative Effects: Dry Mouth (VH), Dry Eyes
    (M), Dizziness (M), Anxiety (L), Paranoia (L)
Reported Treatment Uses: Stress (VH), Pain (VH),
    Insomnia (VH), Depression (M), Muscle Spasms (L)
Description: Grows increasingly purple as approaches harvest.
Growing Hints: Moderately easy grow. Does well both
    indoors and outdoors.
Additional Notes: Very popular.

Notes

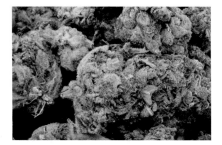

Strain: Grapefruit

Dominance: 70/30 (sativa dominant)
Parent Plants: Cinderella 99 x Unknown sativa
Grower: Multiple breeders
Awards: N/A
THC: 20–25%
CBD: 0.2%
Flowering: 9 to 10 weeks
Yield: 14oz/m2 indoors; 30oz/plant outdoors
Potential Positive Effects: Euphoria (M), Happiness (VH), Creativity (M), Energetic (H)
Potential Negative Effects: Dry Mouth (VH), Dry Eyes (M), Paranoia (VL), Dizziness (VL), Headache (VL)
Reported Treatment Uses: Stress (VH), Pain (M), Depression (VH), Fatigue (M), Headache (M)
Description: Smells and tastes of sweet, tangy grapefruit.
Growing Hints: Very short (3 feet), likes Mediterranean climate.
Additional Notes: Exceptionally popular in Colorado.

Notes

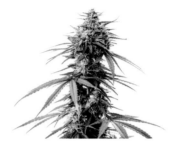

_____

_____

_____

_____

_____

_____

_____

_____

_____

_____

_____

_____

_____

_____

_____

_____

_____

_____

_____

_____

_____

_____

Strain: Grease Monkey

Dominance: 70/30 (indica dominant)
Parent Plants: Gorilla Glue #4 x Cookies & Cream
Grower: Exotic Genetix
Awards: None reported
THC: 25–27%
CBD: 1%
Flowering: 8 to 9 weeks
Yield: Heavy
Potential Positive Effects: Relaxation (H), Euphoria (MH), Happiness (MH), Uplifting (M)
Potential Negative Effects: Dry Mouth (ML), Dry Eyes (L), Dizziness (ExL), Anxiety (ExL), Headaches (ExL)
Reported Treatment Uses: Chronic Pain (MH), Appetite (MH), Nausea (MH), Insomnia (M), Migraines (MH), Inflammation (MH), Stress (MH), Anxiety (M), Depression (ML)
Description: Taste of nutty vanilla and sweet, skunky diesel. Smells like earthy, pungent skunky diesel with a tone of vanilla.
Growing Hints: None listed.
Additional Notes: A "creeper."

Notes

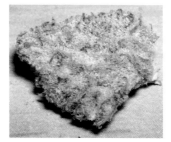

_____
_____
_____
_____
_____
_____
_____
_____
_____
_____
_____
_____
_____
_____
_____
_____
_____
_____

Strain: Green Crack
(a.k.a. Green Cush)

Dominance: 65/35 (sativa dominant)
Parent Plants: Skunk #1 x Unknown Indica
Grower: Cecil C.
Awards: N/A
THC: 12.5–25%
CBD: 0.1%
Flowering: 7 to 8 weeks
Yield: Normal
Potential Positive Effects: Increased Energy (H), Focused (H), Happiness (H), Euphoria (H), Uplifting (H)
Potential Negative Effects: Dry Mouth (M), Dry Eyes (ML), Paranoia (L), Anxiety (L), Dizziness (VL)
Reported Treatment Uses: Stress (H), Anxiety (MH), Depression (MH), Pain (M), Fatigue (M)
Description: Smell is citrusy. Taste is both sweet and tangy, with a lemony aftertaste.
Growing Hints: There are two distinct strains; the sativa-like strain (described here) is by far the most valued (medicinally and recreationally), and you should get a cutting from a known sativa-like phenotype. It can grow up to 12 to 16 feet tall.
Additional Notes: Originally named "Green Cush" but then named "Green Crack" by rapper Snoop Dogg because it hit so instantly and so strongly. It has been changing back steadily to "Green Cush" due to the undesirable association with "crack." Highly valued for both medicinal and recreational use.

Notes

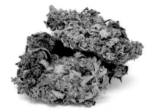

_____

_____

_____

_____

_____

_____

_____

_____

_____

_____

_____

_____

_____

_____

_____

_____

_____

_____

_____

_____

Strain: Green Crack CBD

Dominance: Cross
Parent Plants: Green Crack x California Orange CBD
Grower: Humboldt Seed Organization
Awards: N/A
THC: 19%
CBD: 34%
Flowering: Not reported
Yield: Not reported
Potential Positive Effects: This should provide the same effects and uses as Green Crack (Green Cush), but with a substantial increase in antioxidant effects and strongly mellowing effects from the exceptionally high levels of CBDs and other terpenes.
Potential Negative Effects: See above
Reported Treatment Uses: See above
Description: This is a vape oil (and dispensers) marketed by Heylo and can be ordered from stores in Washington state.
Growing Hints: Not reported.
Additional Notes: Patients who have used this are overwhelmingly positive about its effectiveness.

Notes

Strain: Harlequin

Dominance: 75/25 (sativa dominant)
Parent Plants: Columbian Gold x Nepali Indica x Thai x Swiss Landrace
Grower: Multiple sources
Awards: *High Times* Medical Cannabis Cup winner (CBD/shatter, 2013)
THC: Up to 6%
CBD: (25:1 CBD/THC) to 9%
Flowering: 8 to 10 weeks
Yield: Average to Good
Potential Positive Effects: Focused (M), Relaxation
Potential Negative Effects: Dry Eyes (M), Dry Mouth (H), Dizziness (L), Anxiety (L), Headache (VL)
Reported Treatment Uses: PTSD (H), Pain (H), Stress (H)
Description: Tastes like mango and earthy musk. Very popular with medicinal patients.
Growing Hints: This is a tall plant with a high resistance to disease.
Additional Notes: High CBD to THC levels makes this a very mellow experience. Clear headed relaxation and pain relieve without sedation, causing sleepiness.

Notes

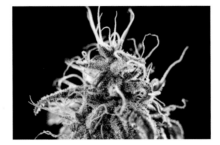

Strain: Headband

Dominance: 60/40 (indica dominant)
Parent Plants: OG Kush x Sour Diesel
Grower: Multiple seed dealers carry Headband
Awards: N/A
THC: 17–27%
CBD: 0.07–0.2%
Flowering: 9 to 10 weeks
Yield: 18oz/m2 indoors; 21oz/plant outdoors
Potential Positive Effects: Euphoria (H), Creativity (M), Relaxation (VH), Creativity (M)
Potential Negative Effects: Dry Mouth (H), Dry Eyes (H), Headache (M), Dizziness (M)
Reported Treatment Uses: Shingles (H), Stress (H), PTSD (H), Depression (H), Pain (MH), Headache (ML)
Description: Tastes and smells like earthy lemon, diesel, and tangy lavender.
Growing Hints: Medium height, prefers Mediterranean climate. Hates frost. Easy grow.
Additional Notes: Smoker feels like head is wrapped and a bit foggy.

Notes

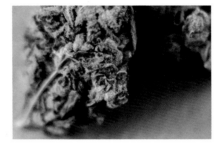

Strain: Herijuana

Dominance: 80/20 (indica dominant)

Parent Plants: Humboldt County Afghan x Petrolia Headstash (bred to the 15th generation)

Grower: Woodhorse Seeds

Awards: Cannabis Cup (best indica, 2015); Jack Herer Cup (best indica, 2016)

THC: 25%

CBD: Not reported

Flowering: 7 to 9 weeks

Yield: 500g/m2 indoors; 500 or more g/plant outdoors

Potential Positive Effects: Relaxation (VH), Euphoria (M), Sleepiness (MH), Happiness (MH)

Potential Negative Effects: Dry Mouth (VH), Dry Eyes (VH), Anxiety (L), Paranoia (M)

Reported Treatment Uses: Stress (VH), Pain (H), Insomnia (VH), Depression (M)

Description: Best for insomnia in LOW doses. Zero activity, excellent for pain.

Growing Hints: Grows like a sativa, but buds quickly and with large buds of an indica.

Additional Notes: Very popular for pain.

Notes

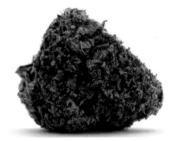

Strain: Hog's Breath
(a.k.a. The Hog)

Dominance: 100% indica
Parent Plants: Hindu Kush Landrace x Afghani Landrace
Grower: "The Hog" of Tennessee. Passed on only in cuttings
Awards: Cannabis Cup winner (best indica, 2002)
THC: 13–23%
CBD: Not reported
Flowering: 7 to 9 weeks
Yield: 400–600g/m2 indoors; similar/plant outdoors
Potential Positive Effects: Energetic (VH), Euphoria (L),
    Creativity (VH), Happiness (L), Relaxation (L)
Potential Negative Effects: Dry Mouth (VH), Headache (H),
    Dry Eyes (VL), Paranoia (VL)
Reported Treatment Uses: Stress (VH), Pain (H),
    Insomnia (HM), Depression (M), Nausea (ML)
Description: Smells and tastes like fruity skunk crossed with
    a wet dog. An acquired taste.
Growing Hints: Easy grow, 4 to 5 feet max.
Additional Notes: Considered ideal for pain. NOT the
    same as Hawgs Breath, which was developed by James
    Hawg in San Diego.

100 Best Cannabis Strains

Notes

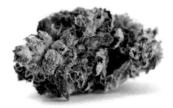

Strain: Jack Frost

Dominance: Sativa-dominant, but % not listed
Parent Plants: Jack Herer x White Widow x Northern Lights #5 x Rainbow Kashmiri
Grower: Goldenseed
Awards: Berkeley Patients Group "All Star" Award (2010)
THC: 16–23%
CBD: Not reported
Flowering: 8 weeks
Yield: 16oz/m2 indoors; 19oz/plant outdoors
Potential Positive Effects: Uplifting, Socializing, Multitasking
Potential Negative Effects: Dry Mouth (M), Dry Eyes (L), Dizziness (L), Anxiety (L), Paranoia (L)
Reported Treatment Uses: Anxiety (H), Stress (H), Sexual Arousal (H), Writer's Block (H), Depression (H), Fatigue (H)
Description: Tastes like earthy, woody pine.
Growing Hints: This plant should *not* be topped.
Additional Notes: No additional notes available.

Notes

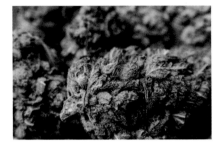

_____
_____
_____
_____
_____
_____
_____
_____
_____
_____
_____
_____
_____
_____
_____
_____
_____
_____
_____
_____
_____

Strain: Jack Herer

Dominance: 55/45 (sativa dominant)
Parent Plants: Haze hybrid x (Northern Lights #5 x Shiva Skunk)
Grower: Sensi Seeds
Awards: Winner of the most awards of any medicinal cannabis strain, including two *High Times* Cannabis Cups and 12 High Life Cups
THC: 18–23%
CBD: <0.1%
Flowering: 7 to 10 weeks
Yield: Extremely high indoors and a little above average outdoors
Potential Positive Effects: Euphoria (H), Happiness (H), Uplifting (H), Creativity (H), Energetic (H), Giggles
Potential Negative Effects: Dry Eyes (L), Dry Mouth (L), Anxiety (VL), Paranoia (VL), Dizziness (VL)
Reported Treatment Uses: Bipolar Disorder, PTSD, Depression, Mood, Pain, Stress, Creativity, Shingles, ADHD, Anxiety, Fatigue
Description: The entire plant—even the stems—are covered in trichomes, making it appear sugar coated.
Growing Hints: Indoors it loves a SCROG setup. An easy grow both indoors and outdoors.
Additional Notes: There are several phenotypes, and the sativa types are most highly prized, but even the indica types are much appreciated. Very popular with both newbies and experienced patients.

Notes

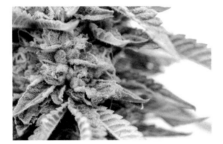

_____
_____
_____
_____
_____
_____
_____
_____
_____
_____
_____
_____
_____
_____
_____
_____
_____
_____
_____
_____
_____

Strain: Jack Horror

Dominance: 70/30 (sativa dominant)
Parent Plants: Northern Lights x Haze x Skunk #1 (a phenotype of Jack Herer)
Grower: Sensi Seeds
Awards: N/A
THC: 15–24%
CBD: Not reported
Flowering: 9 to 11 weeks
Yield: 7oz to 1 lb/m2 indoors; up to 1 lb/plant outdoors
Potential Positive Effects: Euphoria (ExH), Happiness (ExH), Creativity (M), Hungry (M), Relaxation (M)
Potential Negative Effects: Dry Mouth (VH), Dry Eyes (VH), Anxiety (ExL), Dizziness (ExL)
Reported Treatment Uses: Depression (ExH), Stress (VH), Appetite (M), Fatigue (L), Insomnia (L)
Description: Smells earthy, grassy, herbal, and floral. Tastes sweet, spicy, herbal, nutty, and similar to honey candy and berries.
Growing Hints: Prefers a Mediterranean climate, grows to 10 ft outdoors. Growing experience suggested.
Additional Notes: Jack Horror is a play on the name Jack Herer, one of the famous names in the world of cannabis breeders. It is, in fact, a phenotype of the strain Jack Herer. No one has reported on why "horror" was used in the name, but it is famous for the most powerful sense of euphoria of any strain. Take care—one of the strongest of all strains.

Notes

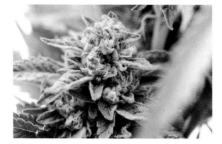

Strain: Jillybean

Dominance: 60/40 (sativa dominant)
Parent Plants: Orange Velvet x Space Queen
Grower: Dark Heart Nursery, developed by Green Avengers
   member Ms. Jill
Awards: N/A
THC: 15–18%
CBD: 1%
Flowering: 9 to 10 weeks
Yield: 8os/m2 indoors; 8 to 12 oz/plant outdoors
Potential Positive Effects: Euphoria (VH), Happiness
   (VH), Uplifting (VH), Creativity (M), Energetic (M)
Potential Negative Effects: Dry Mouth (H), Dry Eyes (M),
   Dizziness (L), Paranoia (VL), Headache (VL)
Reported Treatment Uses: Stress (VH), Depression (H),
   Pain (M), Fatigue (M), Nausea (ML)
Description: Tastes and smells like a handful of jellybeans.
   Citrusy, sweet, tangy, and tropical.
Growing Hints: Highly resistant to mold and mildew. Easy
   grow. Likes warm and dry climates.
Additional Notes: None reported.

Notes

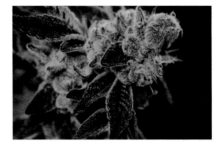

Strain: Laughing Buddha

Dominance: 80/20 (sativa dominant)
Parent Plants: Thai x Jamaican
Grower: Barney's Farm
Awards: Cannabis Cup winner (best sativa, 2003)
THC: 18%
CBD: Not reported
Flowering: 10 to 12 weeks
Yield: 16 to 22oz/m2 indoors; 22oz/plant outdoors
Potential Positive Effects: Giggles, Euphoria
Potential Negative Effects: Dry Eyes (M), Headache (L),
Anxiety (L), Paranoia (L)
Reported Treatment Uses: Stress (H), Depression (H),
Increased Energy (H), Pain (H), Migraines (H)
Description: Smells of fresh, woody, sweet spice.
Growing Hints: Grows equally well both indoors and
outdoors.
Additional Notes: Requires support when flowering for
the heavy colas.

Notes

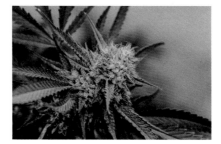

Strain: Love Potion #9

Dominance: 60/40 (indica dominant)
Parent Plants: Northern Lights #5 x Love Potion #5
Grower: Reported as "Unknown Grower"
Awards: N/A
THC: 26%
CBD: 0%
Flowering: Not reported
Yield: Not reported
Potential Positive Effects: Relaxation (VH), Euphoria (H), Happiness (H), Giggles (H)
Potential Negative Effects: Dry Mouth (M), Headache (L), Dizziness (VL), Dry Eyes (VL)
Reported Treatment Uses: Stress (H), Pain (H), Anxiety (MH), Inflammation (M), Appetite (M), Night Terrors (H)
Description: Taste is confusing and delicious, with a milky, sweet, cheesy basis and a hint of sugary mango and grapefruit upon exhale, which sweetens with each smoke. Smell is very similar, with a hint of spicy earth.
Growing Hints: Extremely difficult to find seeds or cuttings of this strain!
Additional Notes: Powerful and immediate onset starting at the back of the head, leaving the smoker instantly stoned and completely couchlocked, followed by creeping euphoria. Creative and uplifted energy follows, with focused motivation that then overcomes the couchlock.

Notes

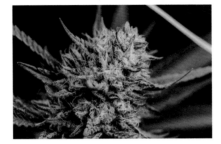

Strain: MAC #1

Dominance: 50/50 hybrid cross
Parent Plants: Backcross of MAC
Grower: Not listed
Awards: N/A
THC: 20–23%
CBD: Not reported
Flowering: Not listed
Yield: Not listed
Potential Positive Effects: Euphoria (H), Happiness (H), Relaxation (H), Creativity (M)
Potential Negative Effects: Dry Mouth (L), Dry Eyes (VL), Dizziness (VL), Paranoia (ExL), Anxiety (ExL)
Reported Treatment Uses: Pain (H), Depression (M), Stress (MH), Anxiety (ML)
Description: Smells and tastes like Sour Diesel with spicy, herbal, and sweet citrus overtones. Has a lingering aftertaste.
Growing Hints: None available.
Additional Notes: Body high with a mental uplift.

Notes

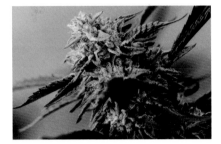

Strain: Mandarin Cookies

Dominance: 70/30 (sativa dominant)
Parent Plants: Forum Cut Cookies x Mandarin Sunset
Grower: Colin Gordon at Ethos Genetics
Awards: *High Times* Top 10 Strains of 2018; multiple
concentrate awards
THC: 19–26%
CBD: 0.08%
Flowering: 8 to 9 weeks
Yield: Not reported
Potential Positive Effects: Happiness (H), Uplifting (H),
Relaxation (H), Euphoria (H), Creativity (M)
Potential Negative Effects: Dry Mouth (M), Dry Eyes (M),
Anxiety (ExL), Headache (ExL)
Reported Treatment Uses: Stress (H), Anxiety (H),
Depression (MH), Pain (M), Insomnia (ML), Migraines
Description: Smells and tastes herbal, peppery with some
citrus traces—like an almond cookie.
Growing Hints: Not reported.
Additional Notes: Calming without couchlock.

Notes

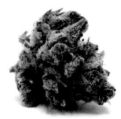

Strain: Master Kush

Dominance: 90/10 (indica dominant)

Parent Plants: Cross of two landrace strains from the Hindu Kush region

Grower: Dutch White Label Seed Co.

Awards: Hydro Cup winner (best indica, 1994) and *High Times* Cannabis Cup winner (best indica, 1994)

THC: 20–24%

CBD: 1%

Flowering: 7 to 9 weeks

Yield: 500g indoors reported. Likely same per plant outdoors (though no reports)

Potential Positive Effects: Relaxation (H), Euphoria (M), Sleepiness (M), Uplifting (ML)

Potential Negative Effects: Dry Mouth (ML), Dry Eyes (ML), Dizzy (VL), Paranoia (VL), Headache (ExL)

Reported Treatment Uses: Stress (M), Pain (M), Anxiety (M), Insomnia (M), Depression (ML)

Description: Balanced mind/body clarity and relaxation without mind-numbing effects.

Growing Hints: Smells earthy, citrusy. Tastes like hash.

Additional Notes: Sharpened awareness making for pleasant activity strain. A favorite strain of rapper Snoop Dogg.

Notes

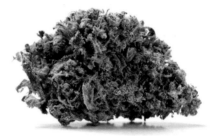

Strain: Maui Wowie

Dominance: Landrace 100% sativa (Hawaiian island of Maui)
Parent Plants: Landrace pure
Grower: Multiple growers
Awards: N/A
THC: 20%
CBD: 0.2%
Flowering: 9 to 11 weeks
Yield: Low
Potential Positive Effects: Uplifting (VH), Happiness (VH), Energetic (VH), Euphoria (VH), Creativity (M)
Potential Negative Effects: Dry Mouth (VH), Dry Eyes (M), Paranoia (L), Anxiety (L), Dizziness (VL)
Reported Treatment Uses: Stress (VH), Pain (M), Depression (VH), Fatigue (M), Headache (ML)
Description: Smells earthy, citrusy, fruity, and sweet. Tastes tropical, like citrus and pineapple.
Growing Hints: This is a tall, easy to grow plant with a very high resistance to mildew.
Additional Notes: One of the three great classic sativas, along with Panama Red and Acapulco Gold.
NOTE: Beware, as many dealers have mixed other strains with this original and call them by the same name, but with different spellings.

Notes

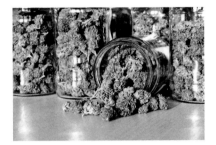

Strain: Mendocino Purps
(a.k.a. The Purps)

Dominance: 60/40 (sativa dominant)
Parent Plants: Secret, not released
Grower: BC Bud Depot
Awards: *High Times* Strain of the Year 2007
THC: Up to 22%
CBD: Not reported
Flowering: 8 to 9 weeks
Yield: No information available
Potential Positive Effects: Euphoria (VH), Happiness (VH), Relaxation (VH), Hungry (MH)
Potential Negative Effects: Dry Mouth (MH), Dry Eyes (L), Headache (VL), Dizziness (ExL), Paranoia (ExL)
Reported Treatment Uses: Stress (VH), Pain (H), Anxiety (H), Depression (MH), Insomnia (M), PTSD (MH), Appetite (M)
Description: Tastes like caramel coffee and woodsy pine.
Growing Hints: 3 to 4 feet indoors; 6 to 8 feet outdoors.
Additional Notes: Loyal following.

Notes

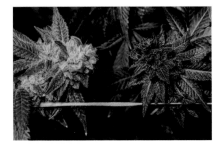

Strain: Mimosa

Dominance: 70/30 (indica dominant)
Parent Plants: Purple Punch x Clementine
Grower: Symbotic Genetics
Awards: 3rd place Santa Cruz Cup third place (indica, 2018); Emerald Cup fourth place (indica, 2018); Emerald Cup 17th place (2017)
THC: 19–27%
CBD: Not reported
Flowering: 8.5 weeks
Yield: Not reported
Potential Positive Effects: Happiness (H), Uplifting (H), Concussions (MH), Energetic (MH), Relaxation (MH)
Potential Negative Effects: Dry Mouth (ML), Dry Eyes (ML), Anxiety (VL), Dizziness (VL), Paranoia (VL)
Reported Treatment Uses: Depression (H), Stress (H), Anxiety (MH), Pain (MH), Fatigue (M), ADHD, Migraines
Description: Tastes and smells like sweet and sour tropical and citrus fruit, with a berry exhale.
Growing Hints: Not reported.
Additional Notes: Perfect early morning pick-me-up.

Notes

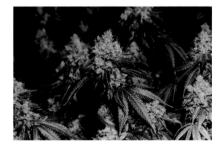

Strain: Motorbreath

Dominance: 70/30 (indica dominant)
Parent Plants: Chemdog x SFV OG Kush
Grower: Pisces Genetics
Awards: *High Times* Cannabis Cup winner (best indica, 2017)
THC: 25.5–28%
CBD: None reported
Flowering: 9 to 10 weeks
Yield: Medium
Potential Positive Effects: Euphoria (ExH), Relaxation (H), Uplifting (MH), Creativity (M)
Potential Negative Effects: Dry Mouth (VH), Dry Eyes (VH), Couchlock (M), Paranoia (L)
Reported Treatment Uses: Cramps (H), Stress (MH), Pain (MH), Depression (M), Inflammation (ML), Insomnia (ML), Appetite (MH)
Description: A diesel flavor and intense smell—as reflected by the name. Hints of lemon, pine, and garlic.
Growing Hints: Only available in feminized seeds. Easy grow.
Additional Notes: Novices beware, as this is a very power-ful strain.

100 Best Cannabis Strains

Notes

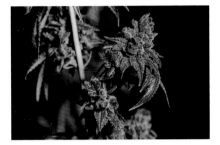

Strain: Mr. Nice
(a.k.a. Mr. Nice Guy)

Dominance: 80/20 (indica dominant)
Parent Plants: Government13 x Hash Plant
Grower: Sensi Seeds
Awards: *High Times* Cannabis Cup winner (best indica, 2008); Glass Cup second place (best indica 2008)
THC: 15–20%
CBD: 1%
Flowering: 5.5 to 7 weeks
Yield: High
Potential Positive Effects: Relaxation (H), Euphoria (H), Sleepiness (MH), Uplifting (MH)
Potential Negative Effects: Dry Mouth (H), Dry Eyes (MH), Dizzy (L), Paranoia (VL), Headache (VL), Hunger (VH)
Reported Treatment Uses: Stress (H), Pain (H), Anxiety (H), Insomnia (MH), Depression (MH), Joint and Muscle Pain (H), Appetite (VH)
Description: Relaxed and mellow.
Growing Hints: Prefers a Mediterranean climate, around 65 to 80 degrees. Does not like rain.
Additional Notes: Named after Oxford graduate and notorious hash smuggler Howard Marks, who wrote his autobiography after leaving prison, entitled *Mr. Nice*.

Notes

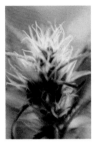

Strain: Northern Lights

Dominance: 95/5 (indica dominant)

Parent Plants: Afghani Landrace x Thai Landrace

Grower: Originated near Seattle, Washington, but propagated by Sensi Seeds in Holland

Awards: Has won more awards than any other strain to date!

THC: 16–19%

CBD: 0.1%

Flowering: 6 to 7 weeks

Yield: 27 to 54 oz/m2

Potential Positive Effects: Euphoria (MH), Sleepiness (M), Uplifting (M)

Potential Negative Effects: Dry Eyes (L), Dizzy (VL), Paranoia (VL), Headache (ExL)

Reported Treatment Uses: Pain (H), Anxiety (H), Insomnia (MH), Depression (M), Relaxation (H)

Description: Even though the THC is listed "only" 16 to 19%, some feel it is the most powerful strain they have ever smoked. Smells and tastes sweet and spicy.

Growing Hints: Under 3 feet tall and considered an easy grow.

Additional Notes: One of the most famous strains of all time. Multiple phenotypes, the most popular two being #5 (which has a shortened flowering time) and #2 (which has the best taste and highest resistance to mold). Now, most material is a result of a cross of #5 and #2 with the best of both, but many dispensaries are selling other phenotypes, so, get the #5 x #2 cross if possible.

Notes

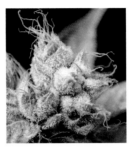

Strain: OG Kush

Dominance: 55/45 (sativa dominant)
Parent Plants: Chemdawg x Hindu Kush
Grower: Many. Originally Matt Berger and Josh D.
Awards: *High Times* Cannabis Cup third place (indica, 2012)
THC: 21–27%
CBD: 0%
Flowering: 8 weeks
Yield: 1 lb/m2 indoors; 1 lb/plant outdoors
Potential Positive Effects: Euphoria (H), Happiness (H), Relaxation (H)
Potential Negative Effects: Dry Mouth (H), Dry Eyes (MH), Paranoia (L), Dizziness (L), Headache (VL)
Reported Treatment Uses: Stress (H), Anxiety (MH), Pain (MH), Depression (M), Insomnia (M), PTSD, Sleep Apnea, Anorexia
Description: Tastes and smells like fuel, skunk, and spice.
Growing Hints: Loves a SCROG setup indoors. If not, be sure to "super crop." Makes the ideal parent plant.
Additional Notes: The first strain to have "OG" added to its name. There are four theories as to what "OG" stands for, the two most popular being "Ocean Grown" (from the Northern California regions overlooking the Pacific Ocean), and the other being "Original Gangster."
NOTE: Many growers mix in Thai Lemon in the breeding, and you will see variation as to the sativa/indica percentages as a result.

Notes

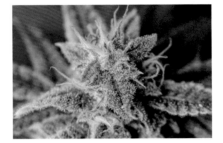

Strain: Orange Tree

Dominance: 60/40 (indica dominant)
Parent Plants: Orange Valley OG x 24K Gold
Grower: Greenline Organics with Greenwolf
Awards: *High Times* Cannabis Cup winner (sativa, 2017)
THC: 19–20%
CBD: Not reported
Flowering: Not reported
Yield: Not reported
Potential Positive Effects: Tingly, Uplifting
Potential Negative Effects: Dry Mouth (ExH), Dry Eyes (MH), Anxiety (ML), Headache (VL), Dizziness (ExL)
Reported Treatment Uses: Insomnia (ExH), Relaxation (ExH), Chronic Pain (H), Anxiety (H), Stress (H), Appetite (M)
Description: Smells like sour pine and woody earth, with hints of spicy herbs. Taste is similar, with a hint of sweet citrus.
Growing Hints: Forest green nugs with frosty trichomes.
Additional Notes: Totally relaxed, but high and peaceful. Can result in absentmindedness.

Notes

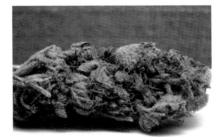

Strain: Orange Crush

Dominance: Indica dominant
Parent Plants: California Orange x Blueberry
Grower: Dutch Passion
Awards: Nor-Cal Cannabis Cup winner
THC: 15–21%
CBD: 0.24%
Flowering: 7 to 9 weeks
Yield: Mid-range
Potential Positive Effects: Euphoria (H), Uplifting (H), Energetic (MH), Relaxation (MH)
Potential Negative Effects: Dry Mouth (H), Dry Eyes (M), Dizzy (VL), Paranoia (VL), Headache (ExL)
Reported Treatment Uses: Stress (H), Depression (H), Anxiety (H), Pain (MH), Fatigue (ML)
Description: Super sweet, tangy flavor. Smells like orange peel and pine, with a hint of berry.
Growing Hints: Grows exceptionally well outdoors, but does well indoors with a SCROG setup. Needs trellis support and central cola pruning, two to three times.
Additional Notes: A good starter strain—not too stoned, but pleasant.

Notes

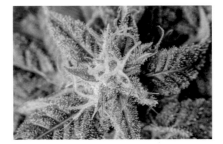

Strain: Panama Red

Dominance: 100% sativa landrace
Parent Plants: Landrace sativa from Central America
Grower: Landrace
Awards: N/A
THC: 16%
CBD: 0.3%
Flowering: 11 to 13 weeks
Yield: 12 to 16oz/m2 indoors; 1 lb+/plant outdoors
Potential Positive Effects: Uplifting (M), Energetic (M), Happiness (HM), Euphoria (M), Creativity, Relaxation
Potential Negative Effects: Dry Mouth (VH)
Reported Treatment Uses: Stress (VH), Fatigue (VH), Depression (M), Pain (M), Fatigue (M), Inflammation (M), Headache (M), Migraine (M)
Description: Tastes sweet, spicy, tropical, citrusy. Smells earthy, citrusy, and herbal.
Growing Hints: Grows over 6 feet tall—not a beginner plant.
Additional Notes: Very popular in the 1960s, not commercially grown due to long flowering time.

Notes

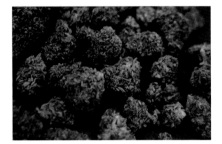

Strain: Pineapple Express

Dominance: 60/40 (sativa dominant)
Parent Plants: Trainwreck x Hawaiian (with several phenotypes)
Grower: Not reported
Awards: None listed
THC: 15–25% (tends toward the lower, 17% most common)
CBD: None listed
Flowering: 8 to 9 weeks
Yield: 18 oz m2 indoors; 19 oz/plant outdoors
Potential Positive Effects: Euphoria (H), Happiness (H), Relaxation (MH), Energized (MH)
Potential Negative Effects: Dry Mouth (M), Dry Eyes (M), Paranoia (L), Dizziness (L), Anxiety (VL)
Reported Treatment Uses: Stress (M), Depression (M), Anxiety (M), Pain (ML), Fatigue (ML)
Description: Smells like pineapple and dank earthiness. Tastes like fresh pineapple and mango.
Growing Hints: While it is an easy grow it prefers temperatures between 70 and 85 degrees (Mediterranean).
Additional Notes: Made famous by the movie of the same name, starring Seth Rogan and James Franco. Both calming and energizing at the same time.

Notes

Strain: Purple Haze

Dominance: 85/15 (sativa dominant)
Parent Plants: Purple Thai x Haze
Grower: Not provided
Awards: One parent of several Cannabis Cup winners
THC: Up to 21%
CBD: Not reported
Flowering: 8 to 9 weeks
Yield: 400 to 500g/m2 indoors; 350g/plant outdoors
Potential Positive Effects: Uplifting (HM), Energized (M), Motivation (H), Creative (M)
Potential Negative Effects: None reported
Reported Treatment Uses: Alzheimer's (H), Stress (H), Depression (H), Pain (H)
Description: Smells like fresh blueberries, tastes like spicy grapes.
Growing Hints: Beautiful purple plant 4 to 5 feet tall. Can grow in northern areas, but thrives best in Mediterranean climates, either indoors or outdoors.
Additional Notes: Named after the 1967 classic song by Jimi Hendrix of the same name, not the other way around.

Notes

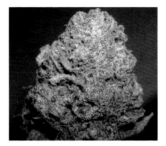

_____
_____
_____
_____
_____
_____
_____
_____
_____
_____
_____
_____
_____
_____
_____
_____
_____
_____
_____
_____

Strain: Purple Kush

Dominance: 75/25 (indica dominant)
Parent Plants: Hindu Kush x Purple Afghani
Grower: Out of the Oakland area in California
Awards: N/A
THC: 15–22%
CBD: Not reported
Flowering: 8 weeks
Yield: Thrives indoors at 400g/m2, but only 100g/plant outdoors
Potential Positive Effects: Relaxation (MH), Sleepiness (M), Happiness (M), Euphoria (M), Hungry (M)
Potential Negative Effects: Dry Mouth (ML), Dry Eyes (L), Paranoia (VL), Dizziness (VL), Headache (ExL)
Reported Treatment Uses: Stress (M), Pain (ML), Insomnia (ML), Anxiety (ML), Depressed Mood (ML)
Description: Smells earthy with sweet grapes. Tastes like earthy red grapes. Small, neon green nugs covered in sticky white trichomes.
Growing Hints: "Clone only" plants grow 2.5 to 3 feet tall. Loves SOG/SCROG setups. Orange/red to rusty red leaves.
Additional Notes: Effects are immediate. Rumors have it there are several phenotypes.

100 Best Cannabis Strains

Notes

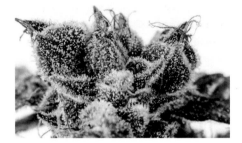

_____
_____
_____
_____
_____
_____
_____
_____
_____
_____
_____
_____
_____
_____
_____
_____
_____
_____
_____

Strain: Purple Monkey Balls

Dominance: 90/10 (indica dominant)
Parent Plants: Granddaddy Purple x Deep Chunk
Grower: Tom Hall
Awards: N/A
THC: 16–19%
CBD: 1%
Flowering: 8 to 9 weeks
Yield: 10 oz/m2 indoors; 17oz/plant outdoors
Potential Positive Effects: Relaxation (ExH), Soothing (H), Euphoria (H), Sleepiness (MH)
Potential Negative Effects: Dry Mouth (VH), Paranoia (L), Anxiety (L), Dry Eyes (VL)
Reported Treatment Uses: Anxiety (H), Relaxation (VH), Stress (VH), Appetite (H), Pain (H), Insomnia (MH), Depression (MH), Giggles (MH), MS (MH)
Description: Smells like woods, fruity, sweet grapes. Tastes sweet.
Growing Hints: Easy grow. Resistant to mold and mildew.
Additional Notes: Great stress relief and relaxation after a stressful day, or a "recovery" weekend.

Notes

Strain: Purple Punch

Dominance: 80/20 (indica dominant)
Parent Plants: Larry OG x Granddaddy Purple
Grower: Supernova Gardens original (also available at Dark Heart Nursery/Emerald Family Farms)
Awards: N/A
THC: 18–20%
CBD: Not reported
Flowering: 7 to 8 weeks
Yield: Medium to High
Potential Positive Effects: Euphoria (M), Relaxation (H), Sleepiness (H), Uplifting (ML)
Potential Negative Effects: Dry Mouth (H), Dry Eyes (H), Dizzy (M), Anxiety (L), Headache (VL)
Reported Treatment Uses: Nausea, Stress (ExH), Anxiety (M), Depression (H), Insomnia (H), Depression (M)
Description: Smells and tastes like grape candy, blueberry muffins, and tart Kool-Aid.
Growing Hints: Beautiful pink leaves with frosty trichomes. Resistant to mold and mites. Needs support, and responds well to pruning.
Additional Notes: Sensation begins between the eyes and then into the arms and legs. Deep relaxation.

Notes

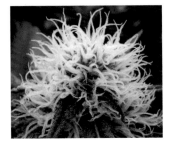

Strain: Purple Urkle

Dominance: 50/50 hybrid cross (though has indica dominant traits)

Parent Plants: A specific phenotype of Mendecino Purps (some say a Granddaddy Purple phenotype)

Grower: Unknown, but originated in California

Awards: N/A

THC: 18–21%

CBD: 0.36%

Flowering: 8 weeks

Yield: About 18oz/m2, or per plant outdoors (though does better indoors in most circumstances)

Potential Positive Effects: Relaxation (VH), Sleepiness (H), Euphoria (H), Hungry (MH)

Potential Negative Effects: Dry Mouth (MH), Dry Eyes (MH), Dizzy (VL), Paranoia (ExL), Headache (ExL)

Reported Treatment Uses: Insomnia (H), Stress (H), Pain (MH), Anxiety (MH), Depression (ML), Relaxation (H)

Description: Smells skunky but tastes like grapes and sweet berries.

Growing Hints: Easy grow both indoors and outdoors.

Additional Notes: Referred to as a "Two-hitter"—meaning no more than two inhales.

Notes

Strain: Queso

Dominance: 65/35 (indica dominant)
Parent Plants: Cheese x Mazar I Sharif
Grower: Kannabia Seeds
Awards: N/A
THC: 13–20%
CBD: Not reported
Flowering: 7 to 9 weeks
Yield: 1 lb/m2 indoors; 17 oz/plant outdoors
Potential Positive Effects: Sleepiness (ExH), Hungry (ExH), Creativity (MH), Euphoria (MH), Focused (MH)
Potential Negative Effects: Dry Mouth (ExH), Paranoia (ExH), Anxiety (M)
Reported Treatment Uses: Fatigue (ExH), Appetite (ExH), Pain (ExH), Stress (VH), Depression (M)
Description: Smells like earthy, pungent, skunky cheese. Tastes like tangy cheese, skunkiness, and earthy.
Growing Hints: Easy grow, grows 3 to 7 feet, likes cold climates.
Additional Notes: Some experienced patients consider this the "best strain I ever smoked." Everyone loves the taste.

Notes

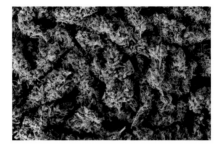

Strain: Rosetta Stone XX

Dominance: Exact % not available, but sativa dominant
Parent Plants: Jack Herer x STS-reversed Cinderella 99
Grower: Brothers Grimm Seeds
Awards: *High Times* Top 10 Marijuana Strains of 2018
THC: 15–20%
CBD: Not reported
Flowering: 8.5 to 10 weeks
Yield: Heavy
Potential Positive Effects: Euphoria (ExH), Energetic (H), Creativity (H)
Potential Negative Effects: Dry Mouth (L), Dry Eyes (L)
Reported Treatment Uses: Nausea (ExH), Creativity (M), Fatigue (H)
Description: Smells like sweet, musky incense. Tastes like Jack Herer strain.
Growing Hints: Vigorous plant with large main collar and required supports each cola. Likes SOG or SCROG, but not required.
Additional Notes: Exceptionally popular strain.

Notes

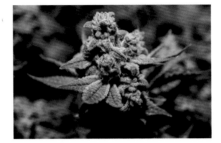

Strain: Santa Maria F8

Dominance: 75/25 (sativa dominant)

Parent Plants: Santa Maria x Mexican Haze x Silver Pearl (then backcrossed four generations)

Grower: No Mercy Seeds

Awards: N/A

THC: 12–14%

CBD: Not reported

Flowering: 8 to 9 weeks

Yield: Very High

Potential Positive Effects: Relaxation, Happiness

Potential Negative Effects: Dry Eyes (H), Dizziness (H), Anxiety (H)

Reported Treatment Uses: Sexual Arousal (H), Stress (H), Depression (H)

Description: Heavy buds make staking a must.

Growing Hints: This plant can be vigorous and grow to a huge bush from well above roof level.

Additional Notes: High rate of negative side effects, reported strong sexual response (the latter of which is limited to the F8 strain). However, for this, the F8 phenotype is a must. It underwent the most extensively hybridized breeding program to date.

100 Best Cannabis Strains

Notes

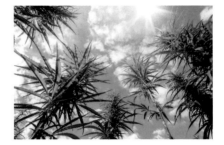

Strain: Sensi Star

Dominance: 70/30 (indica dominant)
Parent Plants: Breeder's Secret
Grower: Paradise Seeds
Awards: Cannabis Cups winner (best indica, 1999, 2000, and 2005)
THC: 20–26%
CBD: 0.07%
Flowering: 8.5 weeks
Yield: 14oz/plant
Potential Positive Effects: Relaxation (MH), Happiness (M), Euphoria (M), Sleepiness (ML), Uplifting (ML)
Potential Negative Effects: Dry Mouth (ML), Dry Eyes (L), Dizziness (VL), Paranoia (VL), Headache (ExL)
Reported Treatment Uses: Stress (MH), Pain (MH), Anxiety (M), Insomnia (ML), Depression (ML)
Description: Smells and tastes like earthy citrus.
Growing Hints: Grows well indoors and outdoors and in hydroponics. Prefers Mediterranean climate.
Additional Notes: Invigorates the mind while relaxing the body.

Notes

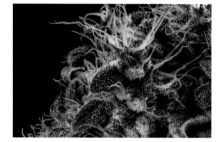

Strain: Silver Haze

Dominance: 90/10 (sativa dominant)
Parent Plants: Skunk #1 x Northern Lights #5 x Haze
Grower: Wherever you can find it, but some "crosses" are
   out there (*not* Ac. Gd.)
Awards: *High Times* Cannabis Cup winner (sativa, 2010)
THC: 20–24%
CBD: 0%
Flowering: 9 to 11 weeks
Yield: 14oz/ m2 indoors, 15oz/plant outdoors
Potential Positive Effects: Euphoria (H), Relaxation (M),
   Socializing, Writer's Block
Potential Negative Effects: Paranoia (M), Dry Mouth (VH),
   Dizziness (M), Anxiety (L)
Reported Treatment Uses: Stress (VH), Anorexia (M),
   Appetite (M), Pain (M), Headaches (L)
Description: Smells of citrus and grass, somewhat pungent.
   Tastes earthy, sweet, and pungent.
Growing Hints: High resistance to mold and mildew,
   medium height plants. Vigorous grower.
Additional Notes: Clear headed feelings of creativity and
   productiveness.

Notes

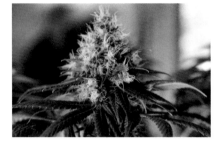

Strain: Skywalker OG

Dominance: 85/15 (indica dominant)
Parent Plants: Skywalker x OG Kush
Grower: Dr. Love Natural Botanicals/Dark Heart Nursery
Awards: Karma Cup 10th place (hybrid, 2018)
THC: 20–30%
CBD: 0.06–0.2%
Flowering: 9 to 10 weeks
Yield: 1 lb/m2 indoors; 28oz/plant outdoors
Potential Positive Effects: Relaxing (VH), Happiness (H), Euphoria (H), Sleepiness (ML)
Potential Negative Effects: Dry Mouth (VH), Dry Eyes (H), Paranoia (L), Anxiety (ExL), Dizziness (ExL)
Reported Treatment Uses: Stress (ExH), Pain (H), Depression (M), Insomnia (M), Appetite (M)
Description: Smells earthy, fruity, pungent, and of sweet spice. Tastes citrusy, fruity, pine, and spicy sweet.
Growing Hints: Likes Mediterranean climate, relatively easy grow, high resistance to diseases.
Additional Notes: Medium tall plant with variable but extremely high THC content. A "heavy hitter," but popular even with beginners.

100 Best Cannabis Strains

Notes

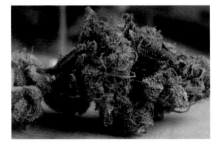

_____
_____
_____
_____
_____
_____
_____
_____
_____
_____
_____
_____
_____
_____
_____
_____
_____
_____
_____

Strain: Sour Diesel

Dominance: 90/10 (sativa dominant). Note: some report as low as 70/30

Parent Plants: Disputed, but generally, sources say Chemdawg 91 x Super Skunk

Grower: Offered by various growers and seed sources

Awards: "100 strains you must try before you die." —*Leafly*

THC: 22–26%

CBD: 0.2–2.0%

Flowering: 9 to 10 weeks

Yield: 18oz/m2 indoors; 25oz/plant outdoors

Potential Positive Effects: Uplifting, Energetic, Happiness, Euphoria, Relaxation

Potential Negative Effects: Dry Mouth (VH), Dry Eyes (M), Paranoia (M), Dizziness (L), Anxiety (VL)

Reported Treatment Uses: Stress (VH), Fatigue (M), Depression (H), Pain (MH), Nausea (M), PTSD (M), ADHD (M), Appetite (M)

Description: Tastes and smells of diesel fuel with a pungent earthiness.

Growing Hints: Most odor during growth of any strain. Grows over 6 feet tall. Prefers warm and sunny Mediterranean climate. Prone to powdery mildew.

Additional Notes: Very popular and available almost everywhere.

Notes

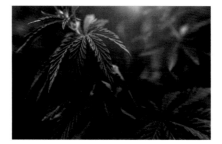

Strain: Sour Strawberry Diesel

Dominance: 75/25 (sativa dominant)

Parent Plants: Sour Strawberry x Turbo Diesel (or Strawberry Cough x Sour Diesel)

Grower: MTG Seeds

Awards: N/A

THC: Up to 28%

CBD: 1%

Flowering: 8 to 9 weeks

Yield: 12 to 14 oz/plant

Potential Positive Effects: Uplifting (VH), Euphoria (VH), Focused, Relaxed, Giggles

Potential Negative Effects: Dry Mouth (VH), Dry Eyes (M), Paranoid (ML), Anxiety (L), Dizziness (ExL)

Reported Treatment Uses: Pain (H), Stress (VH), Inflammation (H), Insomnia (M), Muscle Spasms (H), Sexual Arousal

Description: Smells sweet and spicy with a diesel overtone. Tastes like an earthy, sour strawberry milkshake.

Growing Hints: Chunky green nugs with purple hue covered in sticky trichomes. Prefers Mediterranean climate. Experience to grow: prone to mold and pests.

Additional Notes: Effects are felt immediately. Known to melt away stress and bad moods, often resulting in giggles. Some report increased sexual arousal.

Notes

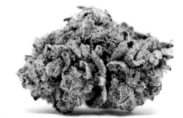

_____

_____

_____

_____

_____

_____

_____

_____

_____

_____

_____

_____

_____

_____

_____

_____

_____

_____

_____

Strain: Strawberry Cough

Dominance: 80/20 (sativa dominant)
Parent Plants: Breeder secret (some say Strawberry Field x Haze)
Grower: Dutch Passion
Awards: *High Times* Cannabis Cup (best flower, 2013)
THC: 20–26%
CBD: 0.2%
Flowering: 9 to 10 weeks
Yield: 14oz/m2 indoors, 14oz/plant outdoors
Potential Positive Effects: Euphoria (H), Relaxed (MH), Energetic (MH)
Potential Negative Effects: Dry Mouth (H), Dry Eyes (H)
Reported Treatment Uses: Stress (VH), Pain (M), Depression (H), PTSD (H), Shingles (M), Nausea (M), Fatigue (M)
Description: Smells earthy with a sweet floral and herbal overtone. Tastes of strawberries.
Growing Hints: Medium height. Loves hot, tropical climates. High resistance to disease.
Additional Notes: Causes giggles.

Notes

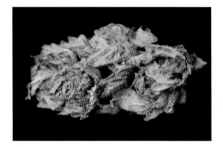

Strain: Super Lemon Hayes

Dominance: 80/20 (sativa dominant)
Parent Plants: Lemon Skunk x Super Silver Haze
Grower: Greenhouse Seeds
Awards: Cannabis Cup winner (2008, 2009)
THC: 22.9%
CBD: Not reported
Flowering: 9 to 10 weeks
Yield: 700/m2 indoors, 1 kg/plant outdoors
Potential Positive Effects: Increased Energy, Appetite
Potential Negative Effects: Anxiety (H), Couchlock (H)
Reported Treatment Uses: Shingles (H), Arthritis (H),
    MS (H), Depression (H), Motivation (H)
Description: Tastes and smells like intense lemon with an
    earthy funk.
Growing Hints: Medium skill level required for a high yield.
Additional Notes: Not for beginners. A "one hit" strain.
    Not for those tending toward anxiety.

Notes

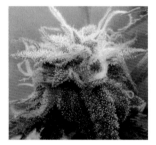

Strain: Super Silver Hayes

Dominance: 75/25 (sativa dominant)
Parent Plants: Skunk x Northern Lights x Haze
Grower: Greenhouse Seeds (bred by Mr. Nice)
Awards: *High Times* Cannabis Cup winner (1997, 1998, 1999)
THC: 22%
CBD: not reported
Flowering: 8 to 12 weeks
Yield: 30 to 130g/plant
Potential Positive Effects: Clarity, Creativity, Energetic
Potential Negative Effects: Dry Mouth (H), Dry Eyes (H)
Reported Treatment Uses: Stress (H), Fatigue (M),
    Relaxation (H)
Description: Tastes sweet and smells of fruity skunkiness.
Growing Hints: Tends to stretch—cut the center stalk for
    branching.
Additional Notes: People like this strain.

Notes

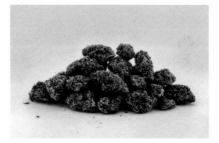

Strain: Tina

Dominance: 70/30 (indica dominant)
Parent Plants: Starbud x Unknown indica
Grower: Constantine x Triple OG (Generation F2)
Awards: *High Times* SoCal Harvest Cup winner (best indica, 2017)
THC: 19–22%
CBD: not available
Flowering: 9 weeks
Yield: Heavy producer
Potential Positive Effects: Euphoria (H), Relaxation (H), Sleepiness (MH)
Potential Negative Effects: Couchlock (H)
Reported Treatment Uses: Chronic Pain (VH), Cramps (H), Inflammation (M), Insomnia (MH),
Description: Smells like acrid jet fuel, earthy, spicy coffee. Tastes like super spicy chocolate with a heavy coffee flavor upon exhale.
Growing Hints: Definitely need to crop this one. Height is, medium tall. Indoors or outdoors OK.
Additional Notes: "Mother Nature's Adderall" starts off with mental rush of enthusiasm, euphoria, and focus, which quickly turns into a sedative, deep relaxation, and eventual sleepiness. Known as the "Thunderdome of Indicas."

Notes

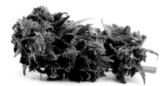

Strain: Trainwreck

Dominance: 80/20 (sativa dominant)
Parent Plants: Tai x Mexican x Afghani
Grower: Humboldt Seeds
Awards: Growers Cup third place (2009)
THC: 18–20%
CBD: 0.02–0.1%
Flowering: Not reported, but outside matures in late October to early November
Yield: 500g/m2 indoors; 700g/plant outdoors
Potential Positive Effects: Euphoria (H), Relaxed (H), Creative (M)
Potential Negative Effects: Dry Mouth (H), Dry Eyes (H), Paranoia, Dizziness (L), Anxiety
Reported Treatment Uses: Stress (VH), Pain (H), Depression (H), PTSD (M), ADHD (M), Bipolar Disorder (M)
Description: Smells and tastes of spicy pine and sweet lemon.
Growing Hints: Tall plant wants warm/dry climate with no frost. High resistance to disease.
Additional Notes: Named in the 1970s by the men who had a train wreck near their grow and had to harvest prematurely to avoid detection.

Notes

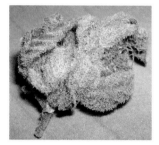

Strain: White Widow

Dominance: 50/50 hybrid cross (Some list as 60/40 indica dominant)

Parent Plants: Indian Lavender x Columbian sativa

Grower: Dutch Passion

Awards: No formal awards listed but is considered a "staple" in Amsterdam coffeeshops

THC: 18–25%

CBD: 0.2%

Flowering: 8 to 9 weeks

Yield: 18 oz/m2 indoors; 21 oz/plant outdoors

Potential Positive Effects: Euphoria (VH), Happiness (VH), Uplifting (H), Relaxation (H), Creativity (MH)

Potential Negative Effects: Dry Mouth (ExH), Dry Eyes (M), Paranoia (ML), Dizziness (ML), Headache (ExL)

Reported Treatment Uses: Stress (ExH), Depression (MH), Pain (MH), Fatigue (M), Insomnia (ML), Migraines, Social Anxiety, Bipolar Disorder

Description: Smells pungent, earthy, spicy, and herbal. Tastes earthy, woody, pungent, sweet, and sugary.

Growing Hints: Medium height. Likes it sunny but does fine in colder climates. Likes a SOG or SCROG setup. Easy grow. Resistant to diseases.

Additional Notes: Considered a "staple" in Amsterdam coffeeshops.

Bibliography

Books and Articles

Americans for Safe Access, *Multiple Sclerosis and Medical Cannabis: An ASA Guide.* Americans for Safe Access Foundation (2013).

Backes, Michael, *Cannabis Pharmacy the Practical Guide to Medical Marijuana.* Elephant Book Company, Ltd. (2014).

Barcott, Bruce & Scherer, Michael, "The Highly Divisive, Curiously Underfunded and Strangely Promising World of Pot Science," *Time,* May 25, 2015.

Bello, Joan, *The Benefits of Marijuana: Physical, Psychological and Spiritual.* Lifeservices Press, Susquehanna, PA (2008).

Conrad, Chris, *Hemp for Health: The Medicinal and Nutritional Uses of Cannabis Sativa.* Healing Arts Press, Rochester, VT (1997).

Danko, Danny, "25 Years of Growing Chem Dog." *High Times,* October 2016.

Danko, Danny, *The Official HIGH TIMES Field Guide to Marijuana Strains.* High Times Books, New York (2010).

Des Barres, Xander, *2014 Cannabis Guide to the Best Strains.* Eternal Bhodi Books, Los Angeles (2013).

J.I. Rodale, *Encyclopedia of Organic Gardening.* Rodale Press, Emmaus, PA (1978).

Grinspoon, Lester, "Marijuana and the Forbidden Medicine," 1997.

J, Sirius, "Highest THCV Strains," *High Times,* January 29, 2015.

Lee, Martin A., *Smoke Signals: A Social History of Marijuana—Medical, Recreational and Scientific.* Scribner Publishing, New York (2012).

"Miss September: Meizy Chiang," *High Times,* September 2015.

McGill, Jenna, *Cannabis: Complete Guide to Medicinal Marijuana as a Holistic Medicine—Medicinal Usage and Health Benefits of Cannabis* (Medical Marijuana for Health. Healing, and Alternative Medicine Book 2). JMW Publishing Company.

Oner, S. T., *Cannabis indica: The Essential Guide to the World's Finest Marijuana Strains Vol. 1*. Green Candy Press, San Francisco (2011).

Oner, S. T., *Cannabis indica: The Essential Guide to the World's Finest Marijuana Strains Vol. 2*. Green Candy Press, San Francisco (2013).

Oner, S. T., *Cannabis indica: The Essential Guide to the World's Finest Marijuana Strains Vol. 3*. Green Candy Press, San Francisco (2013).

Oner, S. T., *Cannabis sativa: The Essential Guide to the World's Finest Marijuana Strains Vol. 1*. Green Candy Press, San Francisco (2012).

Oner, S. T., *Cannabis sativa: The Essential Guide to the World's Finest Marijuana Strains Vol. 2*. Green Candy Press, San Francisco (2013).

Oner, S. T., *Cannabis sativa: The Essential Guide to the World's Finest Marijuana Strains Vol. 3*. Green Candy Press, San Francisco (2014).

Pabon, Richard, *Marijuana and Sex*.

Pabon, Richard, *Marijuana and Autism*.

Potter, Dr. Beverly and Joy, Dan, *The Healing Magic of Cannabis*. Ronin Publishing, Berkeley, CA (1998).

Rough, Lisa, *Do Cannabis-Infused Suppositories Actually Work? We Tried One to Find Out*. Leafly (2017).

Saint Thomans, Sophe, "The Stoner Orgasm," *High Times*, January 2016.

Werner, Clint, *Marijuana: Gateway to Health*. Dachstar Press, San Francisco (2011).

Online Sources

420 magazine: www.420magazine.com

420 Resource: www.420resource.net

All Bud: www.allbud.com

Annunaki Genetics: www.annunakigenetics.com

Blog: www.blog.sfgate.com

Boards Cannabis: www.reddit.com/domain/boards.cannabis.com

Brothers Grimm Seeds: www.brothersgrimmseeds.com

Bud Guru: www.thebudguru.com

Buds and Roses (Carry Joy's Strain, inc. oil): www.budsandrosesla .com

Bud Tender: www.ibudtender.com

Bud Vibes: www.budvibes.com

Cannabis Now magazine: www.cannabisnowmagazine.com

Cannabis Pocket Reference: www.degausspress.com

The Cannabist: www.thecannabist.co

Canna Info: www.cannafo.com

Cannasos.com: www.cannasos.com

CBD Crew: www.cbdcrew.org

Clone Queen Genetics: www.cqdna.com (no longer active)

Culture magazine: www.ireadculture.com

Dark Heart Nursery: www.darkheartnursery.com

Devil's Harvest Seeds: www.thedevilsharvestseeds.com

DNA Genetics: www.dnagenetics.com

Dutch Seeds: www.buydutchseeds.com

EN Seedfinder: www.en.seedfinder.eu

Evolab: www.evolab.com

Gorilla Glue Strains: www.gorillaglue4.com

Grow 4 Me: www.gro4me.com

Grow Marijuana: www.grow-marijuana.com

Harborside Health Center: www.shopharborside.com

Herbal Dispatch: www.herbaldispatch.com

Herbies Headshop: www.herbiesheadshop.com

High Times: www.hightimes.com

How to Grow Marijuana: www.howtogrowmarijuana.com

How to Grow Weed 420: www.howtogrowweed420.com

Hmblt Delivery Devices: www.hmbldt.com/delivery-devices/

I Love Growing Marijuana: www.ilovegrowingmarijuana.com

International Cannagraphic: www.icmag.com

Kind Green Buds: www.kindgreenbuds.com

Kyle Kushman: kylekushman.com

Ladybud: www.ladybud.com

Leafly: www.leafly.com

Marijuana.com: www.marijuana.com

Marijuana Doctors: www.marijuanadoctors.com

Marijuana Growing: www.marijuanagrowing.com

Marijuana Seed Strain Review: www.marijuanaseedstrainreview
.com (URL no longer active)

Mary's Nutritionals: www.marysnutritionals.com/category-s/102
.htm

Medical Jane: www.medicaljane.com

Medical Marijuana Strains: www.medicalmarijuanastrains.com/
strain-guide/

MediReview: medireview.com (URL no longer active)

Michigan Medical Marijuana Association: www.michiganmedical-
marijuana.org

NARCONON: www.narconon.org/drug-information/marijuana-
history.html

National Academies of Sciences, *The Health Effects of Cannabis and Cannabinoids*: www.nap.edu/catalog/24625/the-health-effects-of-cannabis-and-cannabinoids-the-current-state

News THC: www.newsthc.com

The Nug: www.thenug.com

Original Sensible Seeds: www.original-ssc.com

Pot Guide: www.potguide.com

Porter, Nanette, *Canabus Plant Anatomy: Trichomes 101,* Medical Jane: www.medicaljane.com/2017/03/11/trichomes/

Project CBD: www.projectcbd.org

Project CBD: www.projectcbd.org/?utm_source=ZohoCampaigns&utm_campaign=Project+CBD+Newsfeed+%2807-19-2016%29_2016-07-18_1&utm_medium=email

Rhino Seeds: www.cannabis-seeds.co.uk

Royal Queen Seed: www.royalqueenseeds.com

Science Daily: www.sciencedaily.com

Seed Finder: www.en.seedfinder.eu

Southern Humboldt Seed Collective: www.kingofcbdgenetics.com /sohum-seed-genetics

Spirit Smoker: www.spiritsmoker.tumblr.com (URL no longer active)

Sticky Guide: www.91life.stickyguide.com

Strain Brain: www.strainbrain.com

Swami's Medical Marijuana Dispensary: www.swamis420.wordpress.com

THC Finder: www.thcfinder.com

True Herbal Care: www.trueherbalcare.com (URL no longer active)The Weed Blog: www.theweedblog.com

Weed Yard: www.weedyard.com (URL no longer active)

Wikileaf: www.wikileaf.com